"Patrick Daniel provides in_  _usly unanswered questions on ho_ _pro-vides a realistic view of what _ _the many challenges that come _ _ach he shares as well as his pers_ _k to be very enlightening and comforting knowing that someone who faced all the obstacles the author faced could beat the disease. Patrick Daniel presents a thorough analysis of the virus and its impact on your mental, physical, and emotional health before and during treatment. The author empowered me to get in the driver's seat and adopt a proactive stance in working with my physicians and finally facing HCV treatment with confidence."—*CDM, Chicago*

"I went through treatment in 1995 when the only option was the old (non-pegylated) interferon that required three or four (and for some, daily) injections a week. I did that for a full course of treatment but sadly was not successful in eliminating the virus. That was a very difficult ordeal and I have been reluctant to try again since then. After reading Patrick Daniel's *You, Too, Can Beat Hep C!* I have a much better understanding of how current hepatitis C treatment has progressed and what my options are. I now realize I not only have choices that I didn't have before but also that I can converse with my doctors with more knowledge. Of the half dozen books I've read over the years, *You, Too, Can Beat Hep C!* is by far the easiest to comprehend and has given me new hope and a more realistic understanding about my choices for future treatment."—*Susan Z., Sacramento, CA*

"Patrick Daniel's hep C book is exceedingly well researched, skillfully written, and I'm happy to report, quite readable. An exceptionally useful and instructive book, *You, Too, Can Beat Hep C!* will definitely help you avoid a lot of confusion as well as the upsets stemming from all the misinformation that is so easily encountered on the subject. When I first found out I had hep C, it was a nightmare trying to find answers and doctors that were well informed. I have the genotype which has proven quite resistant to the treatments currently available; hence I'm one who has chosen an alternative path. I've two excellent doctors, both traditional and alternative, and judiciously work with both. I sincerely believe my successes are due largely to the research I continue to do, research which has included reading *You, Too, Can Beat Hep C!* I am very grateful to Patrick for his support, his friendship, and for his very up-to-date information. I guarantee that Patrick's book will make it much easier for you to make informed decisions and will save you countless hours of worry and frustration."—*Vicki Leeds (aka Joan)*

"Would you go on an expedition in the Amazon without a tour guide? Or attempt a trek across the desert without the knowledge and equipment it would take to survive? And so you shouldn't attempt hepatitis C treatment without a guide either. Let this quick read, and Mr. Daniel, lead you on your healing journey. This book has all you need to get you through it with just the right amount of comprehensive, down-to-earth, and accurate information. Patrick is a fine example of a man who has turned lemons into lemonade. I now have the privilege of volunteering with Patrick on the Sacramento-area S.T.O.P. Hepatitis Task-Force because we know that people literally, and needlessly, die from lack of knowledge. A book of this nature is long overdue.

Thanks Patrick Daniel!"—*Paul Sousa, CADC Chair, S.T.O.P. Hepatitis Task-Force, counselor Specialist-Public Health, C.O.R.E. Medical Clinic*

"*You, Too, Can Beat Hep C! A Survivor's Guide*, by Patrick Daniel, takes the reader on a journey of the dos and don'ts of living with and treating hepatitis C. Patrick's personal experience is a refreshing, interesting, and often sadly funny account of one man's journey into the depths of living with and being cured of HCV. He seems to have found the Murphy's Law—Anything that can go wrong, will go wrong—method of getting information and treatment in the early days of understanding HCV. Fortunately, Patrick survived, learned copious amounts of information about HCV, developed a positive attitude, and was able to find a path to a cure. Unfortunately, he was not the only one to have these experiences. But, instead of getting cured and forgetting about it, he chose to share his story with others so they may be spared the same misguided path. There are times when one might think "that can't really have happened," but I have heard enough similar accounts, especially in the early days when we were all just finding out about HCV, to know he is telling the truth and speaks from his heart. One of the recurring themes I found so important was the amount of support Patrick sought and gave to others, during and after his treatment. It cannot be stressed enough that we do not have to go it alone and support groups are an indispensable tool. This book is a valuable guide, using a blend of facts, anecdotes from other patients and Patrick's own struggles with hepatitis C, and all of the challenges and rewards of treatment."—*Rose Christensen, Training Coordinator, Hepatitis C Support Project*

YOU, TOO, CAN BEAT HEP C!

A Survivor's Guide

PATRICK DANIEL

Critical Step-by-Step Information For Navigating Your Healing Journey

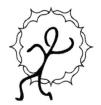

Dancing Dharma Publishing

You, Too, Can Beat Hep C!

Dancing Dharma Publishing

COPYRIGHT © 2013 by Patrick Daniel

First Edition, September, 2013

Cover Art by Jessica Kristie
Typeset by Odyssey Books

Library of Congress: 2013940797

ISBN: 978-0615831787

Published in the United States of America

TABLE OF CONTENTS

In memory of my dear friend Jim Jordan
1948 ~ Christmas day, 2011

I'm not sure if Jim was waiting for Jesus or Santa . . .
probably both

A man of huge heart, crazed merriment, and depth

You are missed

ACKNOWLEDGMENTS

To the benign creative intelligence that moves me forward, often-times in spite of myself. Though it is beyond name, description, and definition, I know it to be that which sustains me on my journey. Never has this been more evident than in these past few years since I decided to be rid of this illness once and for all. It has shown me beyond any doubt that all we need has already been granted, if we can just get out of our own way and accept our gifts with gratitude and whatever level of humility we are able to muster. This is my witness to those gifts and graces afforded me while dancing with this challenging condition and embracing its lessons.

Thanks to Joshua Opperman, PA-C, who directly treated and put up with me during my ordeal. Spencer Baker deserves a special note of gratitude for his support group leadership and being an example of perseverance in the face of great odds. And thank you to all who went through treatment with and shared in the support group experience with me.

A very special thanks to Alan Franciscus for his invaluable assistance in reviewing the manuscript of this book and offering corrections and input. Thanks, Alan, also for allowing me the opportunity to play a small part in supporting your tireless efforts on behalf of the HCV community. A huge thanks to Lucinda Porter for her words of encouragement, support, and a major unexpected endorsement that infused a much needed spark of life into this project. Thanks to Bryan Hill for providing facts and cheerful encouragement.

A big thank you to my dear mother, Danielle Tatigne, for

making this book possible in more ways than one. To Carol, for her support throughout my treatment. To Jacklyn and Adrian, for being there, always. To Bronwyn and Jeff, for providing shelter from the storm. To Michael and Theresa, for friendship and valuable input. To Robert and Lyvonne for loving hand holding when it mattered most. To Jacobus, for guiding me on my maiden voyage speaking about hepatitis C on his radio show, *Gesundheit! With Jacobus*, all three hours' worth. To Chris, for input and sharing his HCV journey; happy healing, brother. To Vicki, for valuable personal insights about alternative treatment options.

Thank you Jessi for your support and helping me connect with Jessica Kristie, my editor and put-all-the-pieces-together lady to make this book a reality. Jessica, you're the best!

Lastly, I wish to thank Dr. X and all who gave me really bad information and misdirection through much of my journey with HCV. Without you this book would not have been possible and others would not have the benefit of my misguided steps. I wish you nothing but the best.

FOREWORD

I have lived with hepatitis C since 1988, and have worked with others who have it since 1998. Many of us are afraid, especially at first. We don't know where to turn and what information to trust. We wonder if hepatitis C treatment is worth doing, considering the risks and side effects. As patients, I believe that we are all looking for one basic thing: strength. For some, strength may mean being cured of hepatitis C, for others it may mean learning how to live with this virus. For nearly everyone, strength means having access to reliable information and support to help us make sound decisions.

You, Too, Can Beat Hep C! offers precisely that—strength. Patrick Daniel writes in a reassuring, humorous manner, with a voice of experience and encouragement. It is as if he is whispering, "If I did this, you can do this too." It is a book I wish I had when confronted with my own hepatitis C diagnosis.

I first met Patrick during a Hepatitis C Support Project event. It was immediately apparent that he had a deep calling to help others with hepatitis C. Although he is not a medical professional, Patrick's credentials are unimpeachable. He knows hepatitis C from the inside. Patrick took a risk, experienced hepatitis C treatment, and is now virus-free.

The timing of *You, Too, Can Beat Hep C!* is perfect. New drugs to treat hepatitis C are expected to be approved in 2014, and multiple options are in the pipeline. For many years, the question was, "Should I get treatment or wait?" Now the question is, "With what should I be treated?" Patrick's words prepare you to be a fearless, well-informed hepatitis C consumer.

Regardless of whether you decide to use the available treatments or wait for the new ones, the reality is that patients need to deal with some of the same treatment-related issues, particularly side effects. I have gone through hepatitis C treatment three times, and although my most recent experience used an interferon-free regimen in a clinical trial setting, side effects demanded my attention. *You, Too, Can Beat Hep C!* prepares you for treatment and equips you with tips for managing side effects, regardless of the medications prescribed for you.

You, Too, Can Beat Hep C! is a highly-readable book. Patrick is unabashedly honest. By sharing his mistakes and triumphs, he offers readers the chance to make better choices. Patrick took a potentially painful experience—hepatitis C and its treatment—and transformed it into a journey. His words light the path, showing me, and you, that we can beat hep C.

Lucinda K. Porter, RN
Author of *Free from Hepatitis C*
and *Hepatitis C One Step at a Time* (September 2013)
LucindaPorterRN.com

INTRODUCTION

Reality check

Hepatitis C, or HCV, is not a mysterious disease that we don't have information about. It's not mysterious at all, but it is a rather complicated disease. Because of its complexity and tendency to affect people in so many different ways, it can go undetected for years or even decades, and has a lot of people unnecessarily confused. Confused and frustrated in trying to find factual information among all the Internet urban-legend-style scare stories and well-meaning people who don't have their facts straight. My goal in making this book available to the HCV community is to cut through what can sometimes be an overwhelming amount of confusion and just plain bad advice. What anyone with HCV really needs is the critical information based on facts that will allow them to make positive healthy decisions about their treatment options.

As you read this book, it will take you step by step through all aspects of getting informed, tested, prepared, and moving forward with the treatment of your choice. We will cover the most up-to-date HCV treatment information that is currently available. I share my own journey detailing how *not* to get treated. That's right; if there was a way to get misinformed and misled, I was right there. Some of it seems almost comical in hindsight but it wasn't so funny when I was spending a large amount of time, money, and energy over a period spanning almost ten years desperately searching for a viable treatment program.

This book is my attempt to spare as many HCV infected

people as possible the misguided steps and misery I experienced. I'm sure many of you reading this have also encountered your fair share of bad advice in your search for solid facts. It's time to get off of the misinformation highway and get the facts you need. My commitment to you is to provide the facts I wish someone had given me from day one of my HCV diagnosis.

Section 1

Clarity in Hindsight

Gaining perspective from the past

My journey with HCV has taken a long and winding route, lasting approximately forty years. Yes, forty years is indeed a long time to labor with an illness, but I didn't even know I had HCV for the first thirty years. The bumpy road trip I'm about to share mainly covers the nine-plus years after my diagnosis where I was seeking and eventually found a cure. It's worth mentioning that once I was finally diagnosed, it helped me understand and shed light on a number of my past health issues.

I had always been very active playing sports, running, hiking, and backpacking well into my fifties. For some unknown reason I was prone to a bewildering lack of reserve energy. I appeared healthy, but couldn't muster any additional get-up-and-go when I really needed it. Putting in a longer day or just keeping up with my co-workers and friends was often a frustrating challenge. On one backpacking trip with a couple of buddies, I pushed myself to go with them on a trek to another fishing lake on our third day out when in hindsight I should have rested at base camp. The following day I was extremely weak and nauseous and they almost had to carry me out. When I look back, I realize that over the course of my backpacking years I was sick for several days after almost every trip. I just didn't connect the dots until later, when I was diagnosed with HCV, that the cause was an overburdened liver that couldn't keep up with the extra physical demands I was asking of my body.

Knowing that I'd spent my entire adult life with a compromised liver helped me understand a number of health issues, but left me with another mystery that highlights the lack of HCV knowledge in the general medical community. What baffled me in looking back was why none of the doctors I consulted over the many years of exploring my energy and stamina challenges never thought to have me tested for HCV. They knew my past history of intravenous drug use and that I had hepatitis B during the same time period, but evidently didn't have the training to put the pieces of the puzzle together.

Maybe your HCV diagnosis has shed light on your past, as mine did for me, or maybe you've always felt pretty okay and still feel fine now. That's the crazy thing about this disease—it affects people in so many different ways and sometimes not at all for a long, long time. It's not called the silent killer for nothing; what we don't know about HCV can definitely hurt us.

Learning from the mistakes of others

Gaining insight into my condition over the past thirty years did nothing to help guide me in dealing with the next ten years of searching for a cure. It was a long trek in a different kind of wilderness, and for a long time in the journey I didn't have anyone to lean on. It would take many years of bad advice and misdirection before finding a roadmap that pointed in a healthy direction.

I have always been a firm believer in learning from the mistakes of others. As Eleanor Roosevelt so succinctly phrased it: "Learn from the mistakes of others, you can't live long enough to make them all yourself." As much as I held that to be true, you'll see from my HCV track record that I unwittingly succeeded in making almost every mistake imaginable.

Here are a few examples of the kinds of misdirection I received to go along with my own short sightedness. Maybe some of these will resonate with your own experiences.

1. I was not properly tested; both the lab tech and my doctor diagnosed me with HCV with only preliminary testing.

2. I believed my doctor's outdated information and made decisions based solely on what he provided.

3. Having had the disease for as long as I had when diagnosed, a liver biopsy was definitely called for, but my doctor did not recommend one at that time. I had also imagined it to be a major and scary procedure.

4. I believed what I wanted to believe and let my own prejudice against traditional medicine cloud my thinking.

5. I thought I could eliminate the virus with natural alternative medicine and was not open to exploring a full range of options. Please note that there are many natural means that support the liver and aid in fighting HCV. But to date there is no evidence that they can eliminate the virus itself.

6. I followed the advice of well-meaning but ill-informed people.

7. I started my first treatment with a doctor who wasn't a specialist in HCV treatment.

8. And like many, I believed the scare stories I found on the internet.

I was diagnosed in 2002, which was not very long ago, but as far as HCV treatment is concerned that was just the beginning of daylight for a lot of the information and advancements that have come forth since, both in treatment and general information. The two-part drug treatment had only been out for three years when I was diagnosed, and a lot of the information that people had was seriously out of date and often even flat out wrong. Even now, there is a staggering amount of the same misinformation still making the rounds and misleading those who are searching for answers about treating HCV.

Pay it forward

I recall one day lamenting to a friend about my botched first attempt at treatment with an ill-informed doctor and wondered why I had to go through such a disappointing waste of time. My friend gave me a grin and simply said, "So you could write about it in your book and save some other poor soul from making the same mistake." Like most of us I've done a lot of things that given the chance to do over, I would gladly do much differently. Maybe we can't time travel to change those outcomes but one thing we can do is share our experiences with others who might find themselves in similar circumstances, hopefully saving them the misfortune of following in our misguided footsteps in the process.

Sit back, take a deep breath, and relax. Know that I've been in your shoes (maybe a slight variation in style and size) and I'm here to provide information that will help you continue on your journey with facts instead of fiction and hope instead of fear.

SECTION 2

JUST THE FACTS . . . PLEASE!

Pass me that Soapbox

Already you've got some indication that I've had some challenging experiences with getting good information in order to make informed treatment decisions. With that in mind please allow me to climb up on my soapbox and get something off my chest early on. And that is that it's just far too easy to get half-baked and misleading information on HCV, even at times from well-meaning sources. We know we've got a challenging situation on our hands when our own family doctors may possibly be included as a source of bad or incomplete information. *How can that be?*, you might wonder. You'd think doctors would be well informed about HCV. Let me ask you this, when was the last time you saw anything in the media about a wide-spread campaign to deal with the HCV epidemic? There are billboards everywhere funded by campaigns to promote awareness of AIDS, cancer, and a number of other conditions. This is a good thing, but I'm still waiting to see one about the need for people to get tested for HCV. So what's the deal? One reason we don't hear much is that of the millions of people who have the disease most of them don't even know it. Too many times it slips right under the radar.

Another factor that stacks the deck against HCV information is that there is a stigma that it's a disease of drug addicts and street people and many institutions would just as soon not deal with them. We do need a wide-spread campaign to educate people who engaged in either at-risk activities or had other potential exposure factors so that they know they should get tested. Those sources of infection will be thoroughly covered in the following pages. It would be wonderful if more people who have been infected didn't have to wait until their liver got so overloaded that it finally called for attention. And sometimes that call isn't too subtle either. There hasn't been a concerted effort to educate either the public or even the health care community.

In the absence of a national awareness campaign we get clinics here and there were doctors, volunteers, and ex-HCV sufferers out of necessity and dedication have become experts in this disease and its treatment. These shining lights offer hope and factual information because they have spent the time to get properly educated.

Med School 101

In med school if you're a Hepatologist you become a liver expert and know how to treat HCV. If you're a GI doctor (gastroenterology specialist) you get a lot of info about the liver as well but not necessarily how to conduct a treatment program for HCV. The rest of the students receive general information about the liver, its functions and diseases, but no real protocol about HCV treatment. Doctors may be informed about what drugs are used, but what to use and how to conduct a successful treatment program can be worlds apart.

Does it have to be this hard?

In my first treatment attempt I ended up with a GI doctor who was inadequately prepared to provide proper information and support to ensure success. I ignorantly stopped treatment half way through, believing I was cured. The treatment should have been successful and I didn't learn why until a year later when I finally received accurate treatment protocol information. It just shouldn't have to be that hard to get information that is readily available. This isn't a secret club, there are no funny handshakes, and you've already paid your dues.

A needle of truth in a haystack of confusion

The statement that the information on treating HCV is readily available needs to be clarified. It's readily available if you know where to look. The information is "out there" but unfortunately so is the misinformation. Misinformation comes in several flavors. Outdated information is one. HCV treatment has only been available for a little over twenty years with many new advancements occurring during that time. As the advancements progress the information lags behind so the public and the majority of medical professionals are left with outdated information to pass along. For instance, up until about fourteen years ago the successful cure rate for HCV was just under 20%. Now with the latest new therapy it's closer to 80% and even higher in some cases. That's a huge difference. Adding to the confusion is the fact that there are several different strains of HCV (genotypes) that also make a substantial difference in treatment and outcome.

If that isn't challenging enough we then throw in the internet, our other major source of misinformation, where there are no filters. During the past few years a number of well-informed concerned individuals, often having gone through the wringer of bad info themselves, have set up some excellent web sites. But there's still a lot of old, misleading, and hyped-up information floating around on the internet. Now that we've identified the problem let's explore some viable solutions.

Get the facts and get informed

If you have HCV and are well informed you are automatically in a position to help others just by the fact that you can point them in a healthy informed direction and counter some of the scare stories they may have fallen prey to. You may even find yourself in the unenviable position of trying to enlighten a medical practitioner who is less than educated on the disease you are seeking his/her help with. If that practitioner is open minded that's great, if not, you're going to have to seek out advice elsewhere.

Some blessed day there may be a vaccine for HCV, but until then anyone who treats HCV, has HCV, or is an advocate for treatment, has to keep informed to stay current on treatment options. Even with a vaccine, that will only take care of the problem moving forward. For the near term there are still the four million plus in the U.S. who are already infected.

Regarding Natural/Alternative treatment options

I don't have a problem of addressing "alternative" treatment options. Just to be clear, I have over thirty-five years of experience being treated by natural/alternative healing methods and living a healthy lifestyle. I am not for or against modern vs. traditional medicine. After trying both I'm just interested in what works. And it's not one size fits all so we will explore both, or a combination of treatment options. Since I'm neither a medical doctor nor a naturopathic doctor, only someone who ended up with HCV, I'm not going to try to convince you to pursue one treatment over another. I will share my experiences, the knowledge I gained in the process, so you can arrive at a place of making an informed decision that you are comfortable with that much quicker.

I used so-called alternative healing methods consisting of vitamins, herbs, and body work exclusively for about seven years until undertaking my first treatment with interferon and ribavirin. The natural means I employed were beneficial in lowering my through-the-roof liver enzymes and helping me with my early symptoms after diagnosis and subsequent nose dive into full blown chronic HCV liver challenges. My high liver enzyme counts were the first indication that my liver was not doing well. While the natural products and therapies I used substantially helped early on, they were not able to cure and eliminate the HCV virus on their own. I believe, and research is proving, that natural products and modalities can be of value in strengthening and supporting your liver and immune system. If you can't, or chose not to do conventional treatment, or are waiting to see what developments are coming in the near future, then I would recommend finding reliable assistance and information towards leading a healthier lifestyle which might include natural products and treatment modalities. The healthier we are in spite of having HCV the less stress and burden is placed on the liver. But as mentioned already, there is no documented cure for eliminating the virus through other means than conventional treatment. I wish it were otherwise and will always keep an open mind. Yes, I've seen the ads on the internet and all I can say is that so-called natural products need to be held to the same stringent testing and procedures as man-made drugs before claiming a "cure." Without before-and-after viral load tests and some serious proof it's all just talk. As with all things in the marketplace, "buyer beware."

I have no agenda except to inform and support those with HCV towards greater health. Since I achieved a cure using the standard drug treatment that will be the main focus of the information I share. Even if your situation by choice or circumstance dictates that you do not use the two (or now three) drug treatments, all of the information will still be valid in helping you make that choice. HCV testing is the key no matter what course you may follow.

Awareness is its own blessing

I often tell new people, and remind us old timers, that this disease can be seen as a blessing if we allow it to take us to its full healing capacity. It will wake us up to our bodies and our responsibility for our own wellbeing. We will no longer be ignorant about all that *stuff* inside our bodies and what it does.

HCV forces us to examine our lives and our health from many new perspectives that we might not otherwise have paid attention to. When we realize how vital, and to a certain degree, how sensitive our liver is, not only to the food and substances we ingest but also to the stress and strain of modern living, we gain new appreciation for taking care of our health and general wellness. Not only can we be cured of HCV, but also, in the process, change our lives, our attitudes, and our diets so that once cured we can avoid many of the lifestyle disasters that are claiming lives at an alarming rate. We're all aware that many of our unhealthy habits, if left uncorrected, can lead to an increased risk of diabetes, heart problems, stroke, cancer, and many other chronic life threatening conditions. Once we go through the process of ridding ourselves of this virus by necessity, we've adopted many new habits that can be of benefit for the rest of our lives.

This message was sponsored by your liver; remember it's the workhorse of your physical body, be kind to it and treat it well and it will serve you faithfully. We don't control near as much as we like to think in life, but we do control our choices.

SECTION 3

MEET YOUR LIVER AND ITS ARCH ENEMY

To deal with HCV effectively we need to have a good understanding of the liver. Being knowledgeable will not only allow us to make decisions that are beneficial towards healing our condition but also help us avoid things that are harmful. Knowing that having HCV is not good is pretty obvious, but knowing that having HCV and understanding what to avoid in order to keep it from getting worst, and acting on that information, is another thing entirely. For instance, by now we've probably figured out that drinking alcohol or taking recreational drugs is kind of like pouring gasoline on a fire when we have HCV. But that just covers one area of concern, a very important one, but by no means the only concern. Along with alcohol and drugs we also want to be aware that a fatty diet, too much sugar, smoking, and other unhealthy habits all add extra stress to the liver. That's why they are unhealthy; they are not easily processed by the liver and that has an adverse effect on our well-being and overall health. Sugar isn't *bad* because it's sweet and tastes good any more than alcohol is *bad* because in moderation it makes us a little high and relaxed. Too much is a burden on even a healthy liver and can lead to serious repercussions over time. And if that is true for those with a healthy liver it is much more important for those with the challenges of HCV.

When we break down the word hepatitis from its Greek origin we find that it defines a condition. "Hepa" means liver (from the Greek, hepar) and "titis" means inflammation. Therefore Hepatitis means an inflammation of the liver. Likewise tonsillitis means inflammation of the tonsils and tendonitis is the inflammation of a tendon. Arthritis is inflammation of the joints, and once again going back to the Greeks, "arthro" means joint. So the point is anything that ends with "itis" means inflammation of that organ or body part.

For purposes of clarification and education it should be understood that hepatitis, an inflamed liver, can be caused by a variety of different factors. Some forms of hepatitis are caused by a virus such as hepatitis A, B, and C, and are contagious. These viral forms of hepatitis are all transmitted from one person to another through an infected substance.

The most prevalent form of hepatitis is not caused by a virus but by ingesting a toxic substance, alcohol. When alcohol is consumed in moderate amounts the liver is able to clear the toxic ingredients from the blood, which is one of its functions, filtering out toxins. When we overindulge in our alcohol intake we get a nasty headache known as a hangover because we ingested more toxins than the liver could filter out, and those toxins are polluting our body's system. Paying a price for too much "fun" is our body's way of alerting us to danger. Our liver, as all aspects of our life, needs things in moderation, and will always try to steer us in that direction. But as a friend of mine is fond of saying, "Earth is a planet of slow learners."

When the liver is compromised and inflamed from the over consumption of alcohol on an ongoing basis, over a period of time, we can develop what is called alcoholic hepatitis. Simply put, the liver becomes inflamed from the burden of trying to process more alcohol than it can handle. As stated, this condition is developed over a sustained period of time. We may be slow learners but we are a persistent bunch.

There is also a condition known as non-alcoholic fatty liver hepatitis, or steatosis in medical terms. While it's still somewhat of a mystery as to the actual cause of this condition it is thought that both obesity and insulin resistance probably have something to do with fat being deposited in the liver.

The workhorse

Within our body is a wondrous system of interconnected functions with each organ playing a vital role. But, when it comes to the task of keeping our body functioning and healthy, the liver is the true workhorse. The liver routinely performs over 500 known functions. Understanding the complexity of the liver's chore list makes it easier to see why HCV affects people in so many different ways. There is a lot more involved in having HCV than just having a nasty virus. The intricate interplay of the virus with not only our liver but also all aspects of our general health and lifestyle all add to the outcome of our symptoms. For instance, I've always been predisposed to digestive challenges and sure enough one of the main problems I've had with HCV is seriously impaired digestion. Remember, the liver produces bile which is an essential part of digesting our food. I would have digestive challenges even if I didn't have the virus. Digestive problems run in my family and are part of my body's make up. Having HCV just makes a challenging genetic situation worst. Our body's strengths and weaknesses, our liver's many functions, and the HCV virus are all thrown together into a big interactive stew. Even though that's a pretty complex stew, we don't need to understand all of it to keep it from boiling over. It's kind of like taking care of our automobiles. We don't need to be a mechanic or engineer to keep up with basic maintenance.

A big part of the "maintenance" of living with HCV is being kind to our liver. For starters, keep in mind the important fact that everything we ingest into our body in any way, shape, or form will make its way to our liver for processing. That includes whatever we eat, drink, inhale, or absorb through the skin. The good stuff and the bad stuff, it all impacts the liver for good or ill. Each of us has a different genetic predisposition to health factors combined with different lifestyles and habits. All these personal factors contribute to why HCV affects people in such a grab bag of different ways. So, let's get familiar with our liver, our body's factory.

A short list of the liver's main functions

- Stores vitamins, sugar, iron, and copper to help give your body energy.

- Controls the production and removal of cholesterol.

- Clears waste products such as drugs, toxins, and other poisonous substances from the blood stream.

- Makes clotting factors that the blood uses to stop excessive bleeding after cuts or injuries.

- Produces immune factors and removes bacteria from the bloodstream to fight infection.

- Produces bile which is stored in the gall bladder and then secreted into the stomach to help with digestion and the absorption of important nutrients.

A closer look at viral hepatitis

We touched upon the fact that hepatitis A, B, and C are all caused by a virus. To keep things simple we'll just say that viruses are very small very nasty critters that are passed from one person to another via a contaminated substance. The common element of hepatitis A, B, and C is that they all adversely affect the liver. Besides that there are more differences than similarities between the three. One important key factor to keep in mind is that there is a vaccine for hepatitis A and B, so it's possible to get a shot and thus be protected against those two viruses. Not so with HCV, at least not at this time.

There's viral hepatitis and then there's HCV

HCV is rarely detected in the early acute stage (first six months). The treatment success rate for clearing the virus in the acute stage is very high but few people are diagnosed until many years later when it has entered the chronic stage (after six months). To add insult to injury, once you go through treatment for HCV and achieve a cure, you are not immune to re-infection in the future. Carelessness gets no slack regarding HCV. Of course, one would hope that after we go through treatment the old ways that got us into the mess in the first place would be avoided like the plague. This is mainly speaking to elective at-risk behavior. Healthcare workers are much more aware and have more protective measures in place today than in days past. And since 1992 the emergency blood supply is now screened for HCV. Here is a tip, if you have HCV, unless you've had hepatitis A or B get vaccinated for them. The reason being that your liver has enough to handle with HCV; you really don't want to get another hepatitis virus on top of that to deal with.

What if there was an epidemic and no-one noticed?

I referred to HCV as an epidemic in the introduction which makes the lack of public awareness even more alarming. There are more than four million people in the U.S. with HCV and approximately one hundred seventy to two hundred million worldwide. For a little perspective there are approximately four times more people with HCV than HIV in the U.S. And we hear plenty about AIDS, not that we shouldn't, but the statistics make the lack of awareness that much more glaring. Here's another way to look at the numbers to show you that you are definitely not alone. Nearly two out of every one hundred people in the U.S. have been exposed to HCV. If given a basic HCV antibody test, they would show positive. Some cleared the virus on their own as will be explained later, so not all have active HCV. But the large majority will carry the virus long term and become chronic. Within the baby boomer demographic the rate is higher at three out of every one hundred. That's correct, about 3% of the baby boomer population in the U.S. has been infected with HCV. I would think that might warrant a billboard or two with some heads-up info for such a large portion of our population.

HCV 101

A patient and persistent enemy

HCV by its nature is not usually diagnosed by overt symptoms because often there are none. Occasionally there may be symptoms in the early stages and some do become very sick as the body attempts to fight off the newly invading virus. But often it's just thought to be a nasty "bug" and let go at that, and sometimes there isn't even that much of a ripple. When the initial infection stage is over it just goes underground, so to speak, slowly invading the body and primarily damaging the liver. The liver actually invites the invasion due to one of its primary functions of filtering and cleaning the blood where the virus is first activated. HCV is a blood to blood borne disease so that's where it starts. The blood of an infected person must come into contact with the blood of another individual for the disease to be transmitted.

Something I picked up in my travels

As I mentioned in the introduction, I had HCV for approximately forty years. Our HCV chronology is usually approximate because unless we had a blood transfusion or very specific incident, many of us picked up the virus along a path of unhealthy behavior. My window was in my late teens to early twenties during my hippie days. Yes, I know I'm dating myself, but since we baby boomers make up a large percentage of the HCV population, this is no place for vanity. Somewhere during that period of my youth I realized I was not exactly on a very productive career path and that maybe, just maybe, I wasn't as smart as I thought. That little glimmer of insight coupled with grace was enough to turn my life around 180 degrees. My exposure time was thus narrowed down to between 1968 and 1972. That personal history gives me a very good idea of how long I had the virus. Plus, in late '68 I had a nasty run-in with hepatitis B from the same activities. I turned as yellow as a lemon and landed in the hospital. I've always thought there might be a relationship between the two forms of hepatitis but since HCV wasn't classified at that time, there is no way to know for sure. Also, I can't discount the small tattoo I got at a flakey tattoo parlor by an old guy who probably didn't even own sterilization equipment. His shop was in a pretty seedy part of town that was full of drug addicts. He was most likely an unwitting one man HCV dispensary. There is just no way to know how many people got HCV from just that one tattoo parlor. And when you think of all the other tattoo parlors across the land, it gets pretty scary. So, you're a baby boomer and you got a tattoo back in the days of fun and games? It may not be a bad idea to get tested.

The question of when and how

A similar story to mine was shared with me by someone I was counseling about his HCV diagnosis. Joe was really straining to figure out when and how he had contracted the virus. We sat together one day and broke it down, eventually narrowing it down to a number of possibilities. The major suspect was a shared needle doing IV drugs with a friend. He explained that it was only a few times and his friend doesn't appear to have HCV now. But we don't know if his friend was infected and he was one of the lucky ones whose immune system was strong enough to self-clear the virus. And there is also the possibility that his friend has the virus but has not been diagnosed. Also, Joe had some tattoos and several ear piercings, which are more minor possibilities. Additionally, as a young man growing up in a rough section of Chicago he had been somewhat of a brawler and later did some amateur boxing, activities that are not short of the potential for sharing blood. Joe engaged in all these activities within the span of several years. I simply pointed out to him that any one of those could have easily been the culprit. How long one has the virus does have a certain bearing on liver health but basic testing is still needed in order to determine the extent of liver damage. Pinpointing the exact time frame is not that important. Roughly ten percent of HCV patients have no idea how or when they were infected.

Often the first thing that happens when we are told we have the HCV virus is to frantically try and figure out how this could have happened to us. That's understandable since the disease usually takes so long to surface that the actions of our youth are often a distant memory. Then there are those who contracted HCV from a blood transfusion or blood products, a dialysis machine, or during the course of health or rescue work, where exposure to blood wasn't considered that dangerous in years past. Again, as far as treating HCV is concerned, how and when we got it is somewhat of a moot point.

HCV transmission: who is at risk & steps for prevention

There is one key factor concerning how HCV is spread: blood. You don't get it by kissing (unless there is blood), you don't usually get it from sex (unless there is blood from both parties), and you don't get it from shaking hands (unless there is blood). I don't care how many episodes of *The Lone Ranger* or *Daniel Boone* you saw as a kid, becoming a "blood brother" with someone who has HCV is not a good idea! Only a microscopic amount of blood is necessary for infection. But there has to be blood, since the blood stream is the first place that the virus invades. From there it can be carried to other organs. For the virus to be transmitted, infected blood has to come in contact with your blood or at least be absorbed into the bloodstream. So if vampires weren't immortal, that would be a good way to . . . okay, never mind that. But you get the idea. The reason this is really important to understand is that if you have HCV, or live with someone who does, you want to keep this in mind. You don't need to be paranoid, just informed and careful.

In an instant everything changed

I met a woman named Linda who attended the same support group as me during my treatment days. She had HCV and a host of other health problems that did not allow her to take the meds to treat the virus. She and her husband Harvey continued to participate in the weekly support group even after finding out Linda couldn't take the treatment. Support is given to help folks with whatever their HCV situation is; it's a condition and experience we all share in common and that in itself gives support and understanding that often cannot be found elsewhere.

Linda and Harvey have been together for a very long time and she had been diagnosed several years prior so they have their routines down and know how to be mindful and careful. Incidentally, Linda was pretty sure she got HCV from using her father's razors to shave her legs as a teenager. It was learned many years later that her father had HCV but didn't know it when Linda was living at home.

One day Linda broke a drinking glass and cut herself while cleaning it up. It was a fairly deep cut, not serious but there was a fair amount of blood. Harvey told her to take care of the cut and he would finish cleaning up. Linda cautioned him to wear rubber gloves as he set about the task of picking up the pieces of glass. The rubber gloves were obviously a good idea but in an instant proved no match for the sharp glass as a piece of bloody glass sliced through poor Harvey's glove and cut his finger. Even though stunned at what had just happened he quickly washed his hands with hot soapy water and then scrubbed the cut with liberal amounts of disinfectant. But to no avail, Harvey tested positive for HCV infection a short time later. Linda was devastated that after all of their caution she had infected her husband. However, they knew from their attendance at our support group that Harvey needed a viral load test to back up the positive finding of the initial antibody test. I'll tell you one thing; there was a big "hurrah" at our group meeting a couple of weeks later when they told us Harvey had self-cleared the virus! As we will cover in coming sections, some people have a strong enough immune system response to clear the virus without any kind of drugs of treatment. Poof, done. We were all relieved at Harvey's good luck and that dear Linda didn't have to carry the additional guilt along with all her other challenges.

A comprehensive list of the most common ways HCV is transmitted

- Recreational IV drug use from sharing needles, cottons, rinse water and any related conditions where unsterilized needles come in contact with shared paraphernalia. This is by and large the leading cause of infection and accounts for about 60% of cases in the U.S. Even injecting drugs one time with shared non-sterilized paraphernalia can be all it takes to become infected. Using a fresh new needle isn't enough if the same syringe, spoon, or anything else is reused. In years past it was estimated that anyone who had been using IV drugs for a year or better had a 90% chance of testing positive for HCV. In more recent years with needle exchange programs and greater awareness of HCV and HIV the infection rates are not as high. The bottom line however is still the same, if one does IV street drugs and shares *any* paraphernalia associated with injection there is a high risk of infection. Some may think that responsible addiction is an oxymoron but in today's atmosphere of needle exchanges and wide spread information on the hazards of sharing "works" it is possible.

    I know a woman whose boyfriend gave her a shot of heroin with his needle one time when she was in college. That was enough to let her know she didn't want to do that ever again and she didn't. But decades later she was diagnosed with HCV and can't think of any other cause.

- Sharing straws or other implements for snorting drugs can also carry the virus as a result of minute tears in the nasal passage. This can be from the straw cutting the nasal passage or the somewhat delicate mucus membrane tearing from repeated reaction to harsh drugs such as cocaine. This obviously takes a big back seat to needle use but still needs to be kept in mind.

- Before 1992 the emergency blood supply was not tested because of the simple fact that HCV had not been classified and recognized as the destructive disease it is. Therefore many people innocently received tainted blood in transfusions during medical procedures. Anyone having received a transfusion before 1992, or blood products (such as plasma) before 1987, would be wise to consider testing for HCV if they have not previously done so. Additionally, anyone receiving organ transplants before the above dates should also be tested.

- It has not been totally verified but there is some suspicion that the air-injected inoculations that were carried out by the military as a faster method to deliver vaccines to new recruits might also have spread the disease. This method is no longer in practice.

- Tattoos, as previously noted, have been linked to the spread of HCV as well. Many tattoo parlors today are fastidious about their sterilization practices, especially since many tattoo artists often use the equipment on themselves. Before the awareness of HCV and other blood born diseases became well known around the tattoo industry, many parlors had lax sanitation practices. And even those who sterilized their equipment would still "double dip" into contaminated ink pots. Don't get a tattoo without talking about these concerns and asking to be shown their sterilization process. Any reputable business will be happy to show how careful they are to promote their establishment. One of the primary ways HCV is spread in prison is from tattoos. Obviously there is not much sterilization going on there! Closely related to prison tattoos are "homemade" tats very prominent among gang members, many who have been in prison where they learned the art. It should be kept in mind that "permanent makeup" is also a tattoo.

- Piercing equipment needs to also be carefully examined. Remember to think "back track." It's not only the business end of the equipment and what comes into contact with you, but anywhere it has come into contact with possible contamination that needs to be considered.

- Personal care facilities such as barber and beauty shops as well as salons that do manicures and pedicures need to also be up to speed on contamination factors, and should be asked about their practices. Make sure that any razor blades are disposed of after each use and cutting implements such as nail clippers and files are not reused without sterilization

- Healthcare workers, phlebotomists, paramedics, and anyone administering first aid or who comes in contact with blood are at risk and need to take extra precautions and be tested periodically. There is much more awareness and training in these fields today than in years past but extra care should always be taken.

- Infants born to infected mothers stand a chance of being infected as a result of blood during delivery as well.

The following are possible means of contamination but are not as prevalent as the above because the risk factors are not as high. None the less, they need to be kept in mind if you are infected or live with someone who is.

- Sharing personal care items with a person who is infected. These include such items as nail clippers and files, scissors that are used for grooming, toothbrushes, razors (blade or electric), and anything that has the potential of cutting, scraping or abrading the skin. Studies have shown that the HCV virus will stay alive outside the body and be infectious anywhere from sixteen hours to four days. Be aware of the potential for infection. Don't, for example, floss or vigorously brush your teeth and then engage in deep kissing a short while later. One needs to think about safety and responsibility, there is no substitute for good common sense. It's also a wise practice to always have a bandage or two in your wallet or purse. Having latex gloves handy is always a good idea in case the need for dealing with blood arises.

- HCV can be transmitted sexually. Among monogamous heterosexual partners it is very rare for sexual transmission to occur. Some research is questioning whether sexual transmission is even a factor within monogamous relationships as long as care is taken to not expose partners to infected blood; the jury is still out on that. Most experts agree that a condom is not required in this situation. However, if rough sex or anal sex is practiced, a condom should be worn as these practices can incur some tearing and possible bleeding. In monogamous homosexuals the risk is higher because of the frequent occurrence of anal sex which can cause bleeding. Again, in this case a condom and extra care should be taken.

- Sexual transmission is highest among those having sex with multiple partners. There is greater risk of exposure with individuals who do not practice safe sex and possibly also engage in at-risk behavior of various types which may include the spread of STD/STI, herpes, HIV, and HBV. The more contact with potential risks of any kind, the more potential for coming into contact with HCV, HIV, or both.

Unfortunately it's not uncommon for at-risk individuals to become co-infected with both diseases. Approximately 40% of those infected with HIV are co-infected with HCV.

SECTION 5

TESTING: FIND OUT WHAT'S REALLY GOING ON

Calling all Baby Boomers

This is what the CDC (Centers for Disease Control, a government agency) has to say about baby boomers (those born in the years spanning 1945 to 1965) and HCV. In 2012 the CDC made the blanket statement that *all* baby boomers should get tested for HCV. The following is taken directly from the CDC website and outlines why they believe this is important.

> "While anyone can get hepatitis C, more than 75% of adults infected are baby boomers, people born from 1945 through 1965. Most people with hepatitis C don't know they are infected."

- Baby boomers are five times more likely to have hepatitis C.

- Liver disease, liver cancer, and deaths from hepatitis C are on the rise.

- The longer people live with hepatitis C, the more likely they are to develop serious, life-threatening liver disease.

- Getting tested can help people learn if they are infected and get them into lifesaving care and treatment.

- Treatments are available that can eliminate the virus from the body and prevent liver damage, cirrhosis, and even liver cancer.

Testing, testing, 1, 2, 3

The only way to get accurate information to make informed decisions is with blood tests and lab reports. Though I didn't realize it at the time (we rarely do) I was trying to make good decisions based on incomplete information. Not only was my info "half baked," I didn't even have the right ingredients. Blood tests and lab reports are your foundation, your primary ingredients that will provide the necessary information to determine what is going on with your liver and the status of your HCV. No matter what you may choose to do with the information from your labs, you can't make good decisions without having some real knowledge about the condition of your liver, and the progression of the disease. Do not let anyone or anything stop you from getting the blood tests you need. Your life, or at the very least the quality of your life, may depend on it. If I sound a bit dramatic here it's because I would have given anything to have had someone set me straight on this one crucial point. I believed a lot of nonsense that I took for fact and spent many years following bad advice. So I admit to being a bit of a zealot with my "get your tests and get informed" mantra.

Facts about testing and understanding lab results

"Oh, by the way, you have HCV!" No prior warning, nothing on the radar, just all of a sudden, seemingly out of the blue, you receive the news. So what led up to this startling discovery? More often than not the revelation comes to us by accident. My personal experience is a fairly common example. There was a bad flu going around and I caught it. I was still not getting well after a couple weeks so I decided to see my doctor. I was due for my yearly physical anyway so he ordered the standard blood work to see if that might shed some light on my slow recovery. The next day my doctor called and said he'd like me to get another blood test. Some of the results from the initial test indicated that further exploration was in order. He didn't mention what alerted him and I didn't think to ask so I came in the next day and had more blood drawn. I was informed that this test was more involved and the lab results would take a few days. Meanwhile my doctor was going out of town for a week so I asked if I could call the lab and get the results, which he agreed to. Considering the test he was ordering, having the lab provide the results was probably not the best decision.

Now this is where it gets interesting and highlights my soap-box about getting good reliable information during all stages of testing, especially the initial tests. I dutifully called the lab a few days later and the lab tech informed me that I had HCV. He said that he would send the results to my doctor so we could discuss it when he got back in the office. I'd had hepatitis B back in my risky behavior days, and had come through that episode intact, so I didn't think that much of the diagnosis. The bliss of ignorance was to be short lived.

We have lift off

The reason my doctor requested the additional test was because my liver enzymes (ALT and AST) were through the roof. ALT was 643 and AST was 412. Different labs use slightly different testing methods but normal levels usually range between zero and forty. Mine had broken free from the launch pad and were definitely calling out for attention. Elevated liver enzymes are a very common initial indicator that there is a problem with the liver. Once that is explored, HCV is often discovered as a result. However, it is possible that one can have severe liver damage and maintain normal or close to normal ALT and AST levels. This is an example of the crazy irregularities that can occur from one case to the next of this disease.

When a knowledgeable doctor is alerted to the possibility of HCV infection with a patient, the first step is to determine if infection has indeed occurred. This is accomplished by using what is called an antibody test. This test will show if there has been exposure to the virus, and was the follow up test my doctor had ordered. This is a relatively inexpensive, fast turnaround test that shows if there are any antibodies in the blood indicating whether exposure has ever occurred. The antibodies tell us that the virus has at some point been present in the body and that the body's immune system recognized the virus and left markers that it had gone into action. On the lab sheet it will state "detected" for HCV. My lab test also showed that I had antibodies for hepatitis B since I had been exposed to that many years prior, and had recovered before it became chronic. Blood work can show antibodies for a wide array of illnesses. The important thing to keep in mind is the detection of antibodies against an illness indicates that a battle was waged; it doesn't tell us who the winner was. What we must keep in mind at this stage of testing is that the antibody test does not give conclusive evidence of active HCV virus in the blood, only that the virus has at one time been present. Most of us do not have much, if any, medical training, so some of these concepts can be a bit confusing. Here's the quick lesson on antibodies. When the body's immune system detects a foreign invader such as a bacteria or a virus, it produces proteins called antibodies, which are used to fight the offending bug. Whether or not the bug is cleared the antibodies remain in the body and can later be detected through a blood test. It's the body's way of keeping a blueprint in case the offending invader returns at a later date. Let's continue with the saga.

The moment of truth, sorta . . . not really

When I met with my doctor a few days later he reiterated that yes, I had HCV and we proceeded from there. But wait, what is wrong with this picture? What is wrong is drawing conclusions without all the necessary information. Diagnosing HCV isn't that complicated but when a vital step is left out the whole process goes south rather quickly. Consequently this is where the wheels fell off the wagon early on in my HCV journey.

Let's get simple

Truthfully this testing process isn't that complicated. There just happens to be one additional test that sometimes gets left out because many don't know that some people self-clear the virus without medical treatment. Often the assumption is made that having the HCV antibody means one has the virus. Let's walk through the facts about testing for HCV. The initial HCV test is to see if an individual has been exposed to the virus and that is all. Remember our friend Harvey who dodged the HCV bullet after he was infected cleaning up the bloody glass? The explanation for his good luck is that approximately 25% of people who are exposed to the HCV virus have a strong enough immune system response to successfully fight off the virus. This is always kind of unbelievable to those of us who have chronic HCV and are exploring treatment options. About a quarter of the people just fight it off, no drug, no years of liver damage. Yes, some do get very sick in the process and some others just blow it off like a case of the sniffles. The actual severity can vary greatly but the point being that in fairly short order they are done and all active virus is gone.

Okay, now back to the antibody test. The antibody test will indicate "detected" for these blessed individuals who self-cleared just the same as it does for the less fortunate 75% who do indeed have the virus. What does this mean to the individual getting this test? It means that a positive "detected" reading needs a follow-up test to see if there is any active virus in the blood. Unfortunately it is sometimes assuming that someone has HCV when all they really know is that the person has been exposed to the virus. And yes, the probability is about 75% in favor of the virus. But this is not something we want to guess at is it? So the next step is to get the conclusive test which is called a "viral load" test. It measures active virus in the blood. If there is any active virus in the blood you have HCV, this is conclusive. Zero virus in the blood, you just dodged a major bullet, you are blessed, be very happy and grateful, and you can show your appreciation to the powers that be by living a more thoughtful and healthy life. Self-clearing the virus is a straightforward affair. Either the body responds to the immune response early on or not at all. Once you've got an active viral load after the initial six months of exposure, you are considered in the chronic stage.

Such a to-do, so much drama

Why don't we just cut to the chase and do the viral load test to start with, and eliminate all the drama and extra testing? That is a really good question. And the answer is that it simply comes down to economics. The initial antibody test is cheap, and quick, whereas the viral load test is very expensive and the results can take up to two weeks to get back. So it makes more economical sense to do the quick test first to see if an individual shows any indication of exposure to the virus. The problem comes into play when doctors confuse detection with absolute infection.

In my case I was pretty sick, my liver enzymes were high, and I had the dubious IV drug history so it wasn't much of a stretch for me to go along with the HCV diagnosis. Six and a half years later I finally got a viral load test when I was preparing for my first HCV treatment program. Wouldn't it have been a hoot if it had turned out I didn't have HCV and my symptoms where from something else? Not too likely in my situation, but it just goes to show you don't diagnose HCV by symptoms, you can only know what's going on for sure at any stage with proper testing.

A recent advancement in the initial antibody testing process has resulted in what is now called a "rapid test" for HCV. Instead of waiting several days for the results, now it only takes twenty minutes. If it's positive, you will then need a viral load test to determine whether or not you have HCV. This test is mostly used at health fairs and by HCV advocates.

Wanna play who has the virus? . . . Hell NO!

Now I'm not suggesting that anyone ever (at least I sure hope not) started treatment who didn't have the virus. Part of the workup to start treatment is a viral load test among a host of other tests. But we shouldn't have to play guessing games after we start the testing process to find out what our HCV status is. And we sure don't want to wait for years until we decide to start treatment to know conclusively whether we have the virus or not. Suppose you'd self-cleared the virus but developed some other condition that had similar symptoms? Be sure you've gotten a viral load test before you accept that you have HCV.

Genotypes and why they matter . . . more "flavors"

After HCV has been confirmed with a viral load test, the next vital piece of information is determining your "genotype" which will be included in the same lab report. A genotype is simply a strain of the HCV virus, a variation on the theme, so to speak. Each genotype has some unique characteristics but they are all still HCV and cause the same level of damage to the liver. In other words, genotype does not affect viral load levels or the progression of liver degeneration leading to fibrosis or cirrhosis. They mainly differ in their response to treatment drugs; some are harder to cure than others. There are six major genotypes of the HCV virus, but of those, only three that primarily show up in the U.S. The local varieties are genotype 1, 2, and 3. Why is it so important to know your genotype? Simply because as far as conventional treatment is concerned, it is the main factor in determining the type of treatment you will receive and also can play a part in the length of treatment, which is no small thing.

Genotype 1

Genotype 1 is the most common form of HCV in the U.S. (and Europe) and accounts for approximately 75% of the HCV cases. It is also the hardest to treat of the three common types. Typical treatment for genotype 1 is now twenty-four to forty-eight weeks. The newer three-drug treatment released in the spring of 2011 accounts for the potentially shorter treatment time. Prior to this protocol the standard time for treating genotype 1 was forty-eight weeks and occasionally even longer. The good news concerning this newer three-drug program is that along with the potential shorter treatment time, the cure rate goes from just under 50% to around 80%. Additionally, for genotype 1s who were not successful with the old two-drug therapy they now have a better chance to clear the virus. A potentially shorter treatment time with greater likelihood of success is welcome news indeed. A lot of genotype 1s who were not successful (about 50%) in clearing the virus are pretty excited and have been waiting several years for this new treatment opportunity. The down side is every additional drug included in the treatment adds more potential side effects. The regimen for taking the third drug is also very tight. It must be taken every seven to nine hours with food without fail. More about that to come.

Genotype 2 & 3, the lesser of evils

Genotype 2 and 3 are often lumped together as their treatment times are identical. There are not that many genotype 3s in the U.S. population with genotype 2 being the more common of the two. Types 2 and 3 generally require twenty-four weeks of treatment, just short of six months, half the time of the old genotype 1 program. These two genotypes have always enjoyed a much higher rate of success (until the new three-drug program came into existence). Of these two, genotype 2 has a slightly higher success rate. With the already high cure rate and shorter treatment time for these two genotypes they are not included in the new three-drug program. In other words, there is no change to their treatment program.

If you have genotype 2 or 3, you count your blessings with humility out of respect for the majority that bear a heavier burden. It's not something you crow about in the support group! I had genotype 2 and give a mighty tip of the hat to my brothers and sisters who had to go through twice the length of treatment that I endured.

The least you need to know

When dealing with HCV it's pretty straightforward what you need to know. First, do you conclusively have HCV? Second, if so what is your genotype? That's it in a nutshell. Everything else gets worked into the equation at some point but these two key pieces of information give you the basic info you need as you move forward with your research and game plan. Without this information under your belt you're shooting in the dark. Way too many people show up for their first HCV support group meeting and don't even know if they've had a viral load test done or what their genotype is. All they know is that somewhere along the line, sometimes many years prior, they were informed that they had HCV. When we explain the testing protocol they often just look confused and wonder why no one ever told them this before, it's very sad. It's fairly simple and straightforward when you know the process, and now you do.

The information you may initially receive may not even be bad, just incomplete. Unfortunately one usually leads to the other. By now you understand why genotype is so important in evaluating and making decisions about your HCV treatment.

I didn't know my genotype and started looking for information on the internet. Right there is a potentially bad combination. With the misinformation I gleaned from the internet and the very sketchy information I had from my family doctor, I went around telling friends that treatment had about a 30% chance of working, lasted a year or better, and made one sicker than a dog with long lasting side effects. That mind set was enough to deter my treatment for almost seven years! And to boot, I had no idea I was running around with stage 4 liver disease (cirrhosis) because no one filled me in on how easy a liver biopsy was and that I should get one. The real kicker was that I had medical insurance when all of this was going on and could have easily gotten the necessary tests and exams. The truth was that being genotype 2 meant I had an 80%-plus chance of a successful cure with a twenty-four week treatment program. I also discovered that a lot of the online side effect information was/is way overblown. Sure, it wasn't a walk in the park, but darn, it was doable! Always remember that you have a right to good, accurate, and factual information in order to make well informed decisions about your treatment.

A completely opposite situation than mine is my friend Joan. Joan runs a successful business and is involved in all kinds of personal and social activities; she's one of the busiest, most active people I know. She runs circles around people half her age. Joan is sixty-three and picked up HCV as I did in the ill-informed days of "sex, drugs, and rock 'n roll." So, she too has had

HCV for a long time. Joan has elected to not get treated. She has a very healthy lifestyle and takes good care of herself. When I first met Joan, as she was sharing all this information with me I was getting very concerned because it sounded so similar to my situation shunning modern medicine in favor of "natural cures." Also, I was really concerned that she was not getting treatment because she felt fine. And as I well knew, some people do feel fine, while their liver is slowly deteriorating and then all of a sudden they don't feel so fine. I was greatly relieved when at the end of our little talk, Joan told me that she gets regular blood tests, and has had a couple of liver biopsies over the years to monitor her condition. Joan may never receive conventional treatment because in her evaluation that may not be the path she chooses. The key factor is that she is staying on top of monitoring her condition and making informed decisions.

I have another friend who upon hearing about my treatment and that I was writing a book confided that he, too, has HCV. We talked for a long time, I shared a lot of info and, like I always do, I asked the basic testing questions. He didn't know if he'd had a viral load test done and of course didn't know his genotype. I asked him to dig in his records and get back to me; I didn't hear back for a long time and called him to follow up. He informed me he was doing some natural treatments and was feeling better. He still doesn't know what condition his liver is in and to be honest, I'm seriously concerned for him. He's following some of the same health choices that Joan is. The difference is obvious, she can back up her choices with labs and facts, and he's shooting in the dark and may just end up shooting himself in the foot.

SECTION 6

IS THERE A DOCTOR IN THE HOUSE?

Finding the medical help you need

If you're reading this book there is a good chance you've been told that you have HCV. By this point you've gained a good understanding of what the tests for HCV are and why they are so important. If there is any doubt in your mind about your prior testing you may want to backtrack using the information in the previous Section to see what tests where actually done. If you don't have copies of the test results you need to contact your doctor(s) and get all of the lab reports regarding your HCV diagnosis. Make sure you always get a copy of any lab reports that your doctor orders. You're entitled to a copy of your labs, but you usually have to request them otherwise they just go in your file. You can also request copies of labs that were done in the past. Don't be intimidated, it's a standard request and your legal right.

You want to be absolutely sure that a viral load test was completed if you've been informed that you have HCV. After the viral load test your doctor would normally go over the results of the test with you and talk about the numbers, what genotype you are, and other pertinent information. If that didn't happen there's a possibility the test wasn't done. If you tested positive for

HCV antibodies and that's the only test your doctor ordered, that tells you that your doctor needs some education on the subject of HCV. Tell your doctor that you want a viral load test done to confirm the results of the antibody test. If the doctor asks why you want a viral load test when he's already told you that you have HCV with only an antibody test, it's time to take a deep breath. Kindly explain that about 25% of folks clear the virus on their own without treatment and you're hoping to be one of them. After the viral load test comes back, if it indicates there is HCV virus in your blood and your doctor hasn't already broached the subject, you need to ask him/her for a referral for someone who treats HCV on a regular basis.

When you're more educated about aspects of diagnosis and treatment that the doctor you're seeking medical advice from, it's a tricky dance. But if they don't treat HCV then they simply may not have ventured past their initial med school training and don't have knowledge of these finer points we're covering. Most family practitioners will readily admit they don't treat HCV and we're not suggesting that they do. We just need to be sure they do the necessary testing that we need in the initial phases of the diagnosis and then refer you to the proper physician for treatment.

Cut some slack

I'll be the first to admit that my own HCV testing and treatment fiascos get me a little worked up at times. Being passionate about getting informed and helping others is fine, we just don't want to get too carried away and start reading the riot act to those we feel should know more than they do. It would be great if those we look to for help were better educated about HCV, especially among the doctors we rely on. Unfortunately, that is not always the case. Just a little heads-up to check our righteous indignation at the door when we work with others who need a little help with the facts. We know there is an education/awareness problem with HCV information. That gives us an opportunity to be part of the solution. As we move forward within these pages you will see that I've had abundant opportunities to practice what I preach. Speaking of which . . .

Stranger than fiction

I sometimes get concerned that people will think I'm making up my bad-info-and-misdirection stories to prove a point. All I can say is that someone must have signed me up for the let's-see-how-long-this-guy-can-get-bad-advice contest. I'm pretty sure I won, or at least tied with some other misdirected souls for first place.

The doctor who administered my first treatment messed up so badly that it's almost funny, but mainly pretty scary. About six and a half years after my diagnosis my energy, and especially my appetite/digestion, went from not so good to pretty bad. I mean we're talking having HCV for right around forty years at this point and somewhere along the way it turned into cirrhosis, so it's no wonder there were symptoms showing up. There is no doubt in my mind that if my life hadn't taken a swift 180 degree turn in my mid-twenties that I would have been in much worse shape and much sooner to boot.

Since my diagnosis I had only been able to work part time mainly due to constant fatigue. In spite of all the natural remedies I was taking and squeaky clean lifestyle I'd maintained over the years, my overall health was still declining. Adding to my dilemma was the prospect of finding a new job looming on the horizon. Being limited to working part time just wasn't providing many viable options for the future so I figured it was time to do something different about my HCV. I asked my general practitioner for a referral and he sent me to a GI (gastroenterology) specialist across town. This fellow, whom I will refer to as Dr. X, treated HCV on an occasional basis and appeared to know his stuff. He ordered most of the right tests (not as thorough as he could have been, so I found out later) including a viral load test (finally getting one!) and a liver biopsy.

Here is where my previous bad information meets Dr. X's lack of proper protocol. The combination of the two was a recipe for a disappointing experience. Part of the problem was my mind set going into treatment. From what I'd gleaned online I was convinced that I only needed to be on treatment for twelve weeks. Hey, sometimes we believe what sounds good to us. Dr. X wasn't really sold on that program but he was willing to let me lead the parade. Not a good thing! I was a deluded patient looking for the shortest cure possible. It was the doctor's job to inform me of the realities of treatment with no wiggle room for wishful thinking.

Home free . . . not so fast!

I started treatment with Dr. X and after twelve weeks I took my first viral load test (it should have been done at week four) and lo and behold I'm virus free, hallelujah! Dr. X asked me if I want to continue treatment or stop. Why would I want to continue, I'm virus free, I'm cured. So many things are wrong with this scenario that it's hard to know where to start. First of all a HCV treatment doctor knows what the treatment time and protocol is for any given genotype and tells the patient that upfront. That's the first reality check that I didn't get. This is no place for fuzzy thinking on anyone's part. My experience has shown that the majority of HCV patients pick up various kinds of erroneous information before finding a knowledgeable doctor. The doctor needs to have a clear understanding that it is his/her job to inform the patient of the available options and lay the ground rules for treatment if that is the chosen path. Everyone needs to be on the same page and committed to a full treatment program, barring any unforeseen circumstances. I came in with bad information and was allowed to leave without being informed in no uncertain terms that it was not the way things work in the "real" world. Three months after completing what turned out to be half of the required treatment time, I took a follow-up viral load test and the virus was back, bummer. It was a full year before I went to another HCV specialist (a hepatologist this time) and found out that the first treatment was so totally lacking in the proper steps and procedures that it left me in absolute shock. After the first treatment fiasco it took two years to work up the gumption to try treatment again.

Time for a little reflection

I think we sometimes go through things for reasons we don't fully understand, until later when we see that it may have served a purpose after all. I believe that life gives us opportunities to grow whether we like it or not. It also gives us opportunities to share our experiences and help others. I take a certain amount of comfort in that. If my sharing this information helps you, then it also helps me to see a better path than self-pity and anger, and in the process practice compassion towards someone such as Dr. X who was incompetent but not malicious. He was older and probably was not up to speed on a lot of the newer developments.

Commitment is the key

Dr. X may have thought that treating HCV was part of what a GI doctor does but didn't see himself or his practice as having that as a major focus. The truth is that treating HCV is a big commitment for a doctor to take on and requires a large investment of time and energy. When done with a "part time" approach it doesn't serve the patient or the doctor well. A doctor who has seriously embraced treating HCV patients will require a serious commitment from his/her patients in return; it's the only way it can work successfully. The other vital part of commitment is that it has to be established early on by both doctor and patient. It's a partnership and everyone needs to know their part in the program. I'm not saying that a doctor who treats HCV can't also be a general practitioner or even have another major focus to his/her practice, only that if they undertake treating HCV, that it be done with a thorough understanding of the commitment involved.

Asking the right questions

If I had the luxury of a time machine this is the checklist of questions I'd make for myself before meeting with a potential treatment doctor. I would literally write this list out and take it with me and explain to the doctor that I need to ask a few questions before entrusting my treatment into their hands. If they know their stuff they will be delighted to have an educated patient who is engaged in the treatment process, after all, as we just said, it is a partnership. If they are uncomfortable or uncooperative about the questions you can figure you're going to be in for some tough sledding and will probably need to look elsewhere for your medical support.

1. Ask about their HCV testing procedure. Just ask the question and allow them to explain. You want to determine if they know to follow an initial antibody test with a viral load test. Another way to go about this is when you tell them you have HCV do they drill down to ask what tests you've had.

2. Do they treat HCV on a regular basis? If so what is their treatment protocol. Just tell them you want a basic idea of what treatment steps they follow and what you need to do before treatment starts.

    a. Do they follow the protocol in the next Section?

    b. Do they conduct weekly or biweekly labs to track blood factors?

    c. Do they conduct weekly or biweekly doctor follow-up visits to see how the patient is doing and to review ongoing lab reports (get a copy for your files)?

3. Do they have or can they recommend a support group?

    a. The 800 number for phone support from the drug company is not sufficient; you need live people if at all possible.

    b. A web site is not sufficient; again, you need live people.

    c. In some cases if you are in a fairly remote part of the country the above two options may have to suffice but at least try to make phone contact with someone who has gone through a successful treatment and who can offer support along the way. If your doctor has treated HCV before, he/she should be able to provide such contacts.

4. Once you have read this book and possibly some others, and have done independent research, you should be well versed in the basics so that you know how things are supposed to proceed should you elect to follow a standard treatment program.

5. There may be slight variations in treatment protocol. For instance, some facilities feel it's okay to test every other week to monitor a patient during treatment. And then adjust to weekly if necessary. Where I was treated they did the reverse, weekly testing and biweekly if results looked okay. Other than minor things of that nature the protocols are well established and a knowledgeable doctor won't mess with the formula.

6. The same holds true with the length of treatment, the norms have been well established. The newer three-drug therapy is more response oriented than the previous two-drug program. In other words, the responses to treatment as measured by blood tests are used to determine the length of treatment. But there are still definite guidelines that will determine the length of the treatment within established time frames.

Keeping things in balance

When searching for a doctor to treat HCV we have to keep several things in mind so that we don't short change ourselves. While we're looking for competent help we don't want to get so fixated on everything being exactly how we imagine it should be, that we lose perspective on certain developing realities. For instance, if a doctor or clinic has been treating HCV patients with the two-drug therapy and appears to be well versed in treatment protocol, do not be surprised if they are not totally up to speed on the newer three-drug treatment. That probably won't be the case, but I'm just cautioning to meet people where they are and not expect more than they can offer. And with new treatment options just around the corner there will be yet more changes in the near future. The clinic where I was treated started their first patient on the three-drug treatment in the fall of 2011. This clinic is in a large city in California and very well connected with large treatment facilities, university medical facilities, and their clinical trials, and has access to a lot of information and support with the new program. That may not be the case everywhere and may take time before some clinics start using that program. Much depends on factors such as the doctors, those administering the program, and their ability to avail themselves of the training they may require. Just be aware that you may need to wait if they are working on those issues, or go elsewhere if they are not able to meet your needs. At this point it's important to keep in mind that the three-drug therapy is still somewhat new territory for practitioners as well as patients. Of course if you are genotypes 2 or 3, that wouldn't be an issue since the new treatment protocol will not be applicable to you anyway. This could very well change soon with the possible use of non-interferon drugs on the horizon. Sometimes there just isn't anyone treating HCV where you live. I've moved twice to get treatment.

For optimal results it's best to keep an open mind as you venture into the process of finding a doctor who will assist you with testing, information gathering, and possibly treatment.

Please understand that just because I've had challenges with some of my past medical practitioners, I don't advocate a confrontational approach to finding a competent doctor. My desire is that you are well armed with facts and knowledge. We don't want to approach this search like an inquisition into their practice. The idea is to be aware and knowledgeable without being condemnatory if they don't meet your needs. There are not that many fully qualified HCV treatment doctors out there. Because of this, I personally found it necessary to pack up and relocate to get treatment, twice.

Section 7

Understanding How Treatment Works

Chemical Warfare

Our own immune system produces a naturally occurring substance called interferon to fight disease. That's the reason why approximately 25% of people who are infected with HCV are able to fight off the virus solely by the strength of their own immune system. Unfortunately for the rest of us, our body doesn't produce enough interferon and/or generate a strong enough immune response to fight off the HCV virus. Scientists were able to produce a synthetic interferon to supply the body with additional fire power, and starting in 1991 it was introduced as the first drug for treating HCV. Interferon is still one of the primary tools in all of the current HCV treatment programs. This may change soon with the advent of positive clinical trials using non-interferon treatment drugs.

The main problem with the early version of the synthesized interferon was that the effectiveness of the drug quickly wore off making it necessary to take injections about three times a week and for some even daily. Keep in mind when we feel lousy from the flu it's because of the interferon that's involved in fighting the bug. So taking it that often was not a fun program. Fortunately a scientific advancement made it possible to extend the effectiveness of the interferon by creating what is called pegylated interferon. This new improved fighting machine only requires one shot per week to do the job. This is the interferon which is used in today's treatment programs. Pegylated interferon not only makes treatment more effective but also more tolerable since the worst of the flu-like symptoms usually last for a day or two after the injection and then taper off until the next dose. This was a real boost to those attempting to hold down a job while undergoing treatment. Some people find that they can take their shot on Friday and have the weekend to rest before the next work week. This isn't to say that you're going to feel great at work because you very well might not, but it gives a better chance of making it through the week.

Another arrow in the quiver

In 1999 the antiviral drug ribavirin was added to the treatment program to make interferon even more effective. To this day it's not totally understood how ribavirin interacts with interferon to increase the cure rate, but it does. Of course each new drug brings its own "good news/bad news" package. Along with its benefits each additional drug brings other potential side effects into play.

The long awaited third drug

The latest drugs introduced into conventional treatment are protease inhibitors that go by the names of boceprevir and telaprevir. The primary function of the protease inhibitors is to greatly slow down the rate at which the HCV virus is able to multiply and replicate itself. With a lower level of virus in the system the interferon and ribavirin are more effectively able to completely remove the virus. These drugs were approved in late spring of 2011 and are only used to treat genotype 1. The three-drug therapy has been long awaited especially by those genotype 1s who did not respond to treatment with the two-drug therapy. Clinical trials have shown a high rate of success with this previously unsuccessful group, giving many people new hope for a cure. Improvement from the previous approximately 50% cure rate have gone up as high as 80% with the addition of the new drugs. Along with increasing the rate of treatment success, this new three-drug cocktail also has the potential for a shorter treatment time. As previously mentioned, the protease inhibitors do present a treatment challenge due to the need of sustaining minimal drug levels in the body. This in turn requires a very tight dosage schedule. If a sustained level is not maintained the virus can quickly build immunity to the drug, thereby nullifying any potential benefit and may even inhibit future treatment. It's pretty much a one shot deal not allowing for a lot of lee way. The pill form of the drug must be taken every seven to nine hours without fail. The side effects of these new drugs can be quite severe for some folks and there are rapid advances to switch to more tolerable drugs currently undergoing clinical trials.

How long, Oh Lord?

The standard treatment time for genotype 1 using the two-part program (interferon and ribavirin only) has been forty-eight weeks. Previously it was mentioned that the newer three-drug program for genotype 1 is more of a response based program. Meaning that the length of time for the treatment will be determined in part by the patient's response to the drugs and what the subsequent test results show. In many cases the length of treatment will be shorter than the previous forty-eight weeks that the two-drug program required. Clinical trials have shown that treatment time can be as short as twenty-four weeks for some individuals. At this point the general guideline going into treatment is to figure between twenty-four and forty-eight weeks of treatment. As this book is preparing for publication there are clinical trials underway that have achieved successful treatment in as short as twelve weeks and are exploring treatment times of only eight weeks.

While genotype 1 patients are undergoing a fairly radical change in their approach to treatment, genotype 2s and 3s as previously mentioned are continuing the same treatment protocol as before. They will continue to use the two-drug therapy with a twenty-four week treatment time. But, with the new advances that may change fairly soon.

Tracking treatment success

To monitor the amount of virus in the blood a viral load test is conducted just before treatment starts to establish a baseline. Then as treatment progresses additional viral load tests are conducted at four-week intervals to determine the effectiveness of treatment. So that's a test at week four, eight, and twelve. Once the viral load is zero, usually no more viral load tests are done until the end of treatment (however some clinics will do another viral load test during treatment to be sure that the level continues to be zero). The purpose of this four week interval viral load tests is to gauge how effective the drugs are working towards clearing the virus. Ideally the viral load will be zero during the first three months (twelve weeks) of treatment. The sooner the virus is cleared the greater chance of a successful treatment there is.

The Early Virological Response advantage

There is one treatment response that tends to alter all the previous cure percentages significantly. This occurs when a patient has cleared the virus at the first viral load test after starting treatment at the four week mark. Clearing the virus at that time is called an early virological response or EVR for short. The good news for those who achieve an EVR, meaning no detectable viral load during the first four weeks of treatment, is that cure rates shoots up to 90%-plus, and that also includes genotype 1. EVR will also be a significant factor, possibly allowing for shorter treatment duration for those undergoing the three-drug therapy.

Zero viral load . . . all done . . . NO!

Okay, so you've achieved an EVR, nice, but are you done? During support group Q&A this is the place where everyone goes, wait a minute, if you're virus free, no viral load, at the end of four or even eight or twelve weeks, why bother going through the rest of the treatment? That's a question I wished I'd known the answer to before stopping my first treatment at twelve weeks. As you may recall I was virus free at the end of three months. The truth was that I was probably virus free long before that but my doctor (bless his incompetent heart) didn't test any sooner than that. Since I was an early responder the second time around with treatment, there's a good chance I was the first time as well.

Going where no virus has gone before

Just because HCV is a blood borne disease doesn't mean it can't go anywhere else. Here is an important bit of information to keep in mind regarding how the HCV virus works in the body, which was something else I was not told beforehand. A viral load test only measures virus in the blood, after all, it is a blood test. Okay, that makes sense but the problem is that the virus is not limited to the blood stream. Since we know it has saturated the liver we understand it can spread throughout the body. Not only is it hard to kill, and replicates like crazy, but it's also really good at hiding out. So this necessitates a pretty big workaround. From clinical trials and firsthand experience HCV specialists were able to determine the success rates and treatment times for the different genotype groups. Stay with me, we're getting to the answer of why to continue treatment after clearing the virus; it just takes a bit of explaining.

Doing the work around boogie

This comes up so often in the support group that I've broken it down into steps so that it's as clear as possible. Here we go, take notes, there will be a test (pun intended).

1. A viral load test is taken before starting treatment to establish a baseline of viral load count.

2. Another viral load test is taken every four weeks (up to week twelve) during treatment until the viral load is zero to see how effective the drugs are and establish a time when the virus is cleared.

3. At the end of treatment another viral load test is conducted to be sure that everything is still clear before calling it good.

4. Finally, in order to tell if the virus has been cleared from its little hidey places in the body, a final viral load test is done six months after the end of treatment. When this final viral load test result comes back stating there is still zero viral load, we have achieved what is called a sustained virological response (SVR). In other words you can then say you are cured. The good news is that it is rare for the virus to come back at this stage, which makes the six month waiting period a bit more bearable. However, I must admit those last few weeks before the six month test is due, combined with the waiting period for the results to come back, can produce some anxiety.

Why the six month waiting period?

Let's look at why we need to take a final viral load test six months after the end of treatment before we can claim a cure. Remember, the viral load test only measures virus in the blood and the virus is not limited to the blood. Waiting for six months allows any residue from the treatment drugs to get flushed out, leaving the body to fend for itself. Due to the rapid reproduction rate of the virus, if there was any virus remaining it would show up in the blood at the six month test. So that's the long answer to a short question. The reason for my first treatment failure was simply that I didn't do the treatment long enough. There was still virus that lingered outside the blood stream and it came roaring back to full glory by the next viral load test. To make matters worse, I later found out that cutting my ribavirin dose in half because of the digestion problems might have also played a part in lessening the effectiveness of the treatment.

What does Non-Responder mean?

The flip side of the early responder is the non-responder or minimal responder. As I'm writing this about two years into the three-drug treatment there will be some possible major changes in the future because results will be different with genotype 1 than they have been in the past. Up until now the harder-to-treat genotype 1 sometimes did not respond to the conventional two-drug therapy and if a significant viral load drop did not occur by the third viral load test taken at week twelve, it was usually figured that treatment was not going to be successful for them. With no or very little sign of improvement after three months there was no sense in going through an additional nine-month-long ordeal with very little chance of a cure. In fact the success rate of genotype 1s who did continue with treatment as a non-responder was about 1%. Over the past several years the mantra for these folks has been "wait for the clinical trials to end and try again with the three-drug program." So now those folks are getting a second chance at treatment with a much higher chance of success. Since there are no guarantees with any treatment there will be some who do not respond to the three-drug treatment as there will be genotype 2s and 3s who do not respond to their treatment as well. With 2s and 3s those are pretty rare; we hope the same is true with genotype 1s and the new three-drug program as well as any future treatment programs.

Understanding the weekly (or biweekly) blood tests

We now understand that the HCV virus is a nasty, tenacious little critter that multiplies at a rapid rate and does not go down without a fight. The peg interferon/ribavirin combination along with the newer protease inhibitors are all heavy duty drugs used to fight this heavy duty virus. This battle puts a major strain on the blood and its ability to function normally. Let's take a look at how treatment affects the blood and why it needs to be monitored on a regular basis.

Red and white blood cell counts tend to drop in the early stages of treatment and need to be monitored to insure that they do not get so low as to cause potential health problems. Blood platelet counts are also susceptible and need monitoring. Prior to starting treatment, tests are ordered to establish a baseline for all three of these blood factors. This will help your doctor to see how your blood counts compare to what has been established as a normal range. Blood will then be monitored on a weekly or biweekly basis to see how the drugs are affecting the levels. HCV specialists have established a minimal count level for each blood factor, that if reached, will necessitate corrective measures or possibly stopping treatment altogether. At no time is the patient allowed to be in danger for the sake of completing treatment. This is all necessitated by the vital functions that each of these three blood components performs. Here is the breakdown of each blood factor's function.

- The white blood cells primary activity is to fight infection. If the white blood cell count gets too low there is the possibility of the body not being able to respond adequately to what would be an otherwise minor incident. If the body is compromised in its ability to fight infection, something like the flu or a tooth abscess can become life threatening.

- Red blood cells carry oxygen to the blood. If there is not enough oxygen it will cause fatigue. Fatigue is already a factor with a lot of HCV sufferers so it's important to not allow the situation to worsen beyond a tolerable limit.

- Platelets allow the blood to clot. Lab reports can provide a means to see that platelet counts are maintained at safe levels to insure that something like a minor cut doesn't turn into a major problem.

Safety fist

Since we know that interferon and ribavirin have an effect on these blood factors the labs help track what is happening and allow the doctor to make sure treatment is proceeding safely. If any of these factors become too low, your doctor will talk to you about possible drugs to counter the effects, or possibly halting treatment all together.

A blessing in disguise

A person in our support group who was not in the best of health to start with was having her blood monitored closely. At one point during treatment her white blood count got dangerously low and she had to stop treatment. She was genotype 1 with about nine months of treatment already completed. Because she had completed so much of the treatment and had the good fortune to be an early responder (cleared the virus in the first four weeks) it was decided to stop treatment and see what her viral load looked like after six months. It was a nerve wracking six month wait for her, but when the final viral load came back clear it was a happy day. She had achieved a cure two and a half months early. A challenge had turned into a blessing even if it was a fairly anxious one.

Keeping the bugs at bay

The situations and side effects presented in these many lists are possibilities of what may be encountered during treatment. Since we don't know what will actually show up for any given individual, think of this as reference material. The information is here to help you be prepared and to guide you if needed. With that in mind, here's another list.

Tips for minimizing your exposure to infection and avoiding complications during treatment.

- Just being conscious and cautious regarding possible exposure to contagious diseases and infections is the first step.

- There is no substitute for good hygiene especially during cold/flu season. Guys, it's okay to get a little retentive and do that stuff your mothers and lady friends always bug you about, like washing your hands often, especially when using public restrooms. And by washing we're not talking running your hands under water so it looks like you're washing your hands, but a good fifteen to twenty second scrub. There is less concern about handling your own plumbing, than the various handles that everyone else has touched (door, toilet, sink, paper towel dispenser, etc.). Many public restroom functions are now sensor activated, but still try not to touch anything after washing your hands. Chuck that paper towel after you open the door with it. This may sound over the top, but the medical community says that is the most important thing we can do when a lot of people are running around sick. We can't live in a bubble, but we don't have to invite trouble in either.

- Most likely your doctor will order a flu shot as part of the pre-treatment work up if any part of the treatment is to occur during flu season. In any case, try to avoid large crowds and gatherings, especially in tight quarters. Hang back and see just how packed that elevator is going to be before committing, especially if someone is clutching a hanky with a red nose and has "flu" written across their forehead. Better yet, if you've got the energy take the stairs.

- Holiday gatherings need to really be assessed for your protection. A large family get-together in a house can get pretty cozy (a hug from Auntie Rose who has the sniffles is not a good idea). My second month of treatment coincided with the Christmas season and invitations to family gatherings. I come from a family of serious huggers; when my white blood cell count was getting quite low during a two week period, it was easier to bow out entirely instead of wearing a "do not hug me" sign.

- Let family and friends know ahead of time that you may encounter some challenges and limitations to your social interactions. Low white cell count or not, you just may not feel up to hanging out with people if you feel crappy. A *heads up* early on might make such situations a bit less awkward. To be clear, I'm not suggesting that you chuck all human contact or family gathering during treatment. The suggestion only applies if you don't feel up to attending gatherings anyway and secondly if your white blood cell counts are heading south and your doctor has called that to your attention. Going through treatment in the middle of cold/flu season always warrants extra attention.

- Not to be used too excessively, but a "medical excuse" may come in handy at times. Sometimes there can be a fair amount of pressure to socialize exerted by well-meaning relatives and friends. They mean well but might be lacking in their understanding of how treatment is kicking your butt. It's sometimes easier to bow out by blaming it on your "doctor's orders" than spend a lot of time trying to educate people who don't get that you just aren't up to joining in the fun and games.

- When not feeling well (before or during treatment) it can be annoying to hear people say something like, "It can't be that bad, you don't *look* sick." Keep in mind some people have a hard time believing you're sick unless you look sick. Most people don't know enough about the liver and HCV to understand the severity of what you're dealing with. Try to gently explain that you don't want to wait until you turn yellow and are half dead before you start treatment.

This is NOT how treatment works

Let's go back to the fiasco of my first treatment for a moment. Now that you have an idea of what to look for in a treatment program let me share what the protocol was in my first unsuccessful treatment. I was given a DVD supplied by the drug company that makes interferon and ribavirin. This is a very good DVD and useful as part of a good educational program to prepare for treatment. But just a DVD by itself is not adequate. I was shown how to inject myself by a doctor's assistant and told that I would get a blood test after one month and a viral load test at the end of three months. At the time that seemed adequate. It was only later on when I conferred with an HCV specialist and attended a support group that I found out how seriously lacking the information and protocol were during my first treatment attempt. Sometimes it's only by comparison that we truly understand and appreciate a properly administered program.

I have to tell this little story just because it illustrates what can happen when people are not fully engaged and working in an environment where treatment is just a marginal part of the practice. The assistant who was showing me how to inject the interferon took the opportunity to train a new assistant on how to give injections. It really should have been, "this is not how to give injections!" First off, after swabbing an area of my thigh with an alcohol wipe she missed the spot by at least two inches from where any alcohol had actually been applied. She also failed to turn the syringe upside down and squirt out any air bubbles and excess interferon. The dose is 180ml but the syringe is overfilled a bit to allow for clearing air bubbles. But no, none of that, she just shot all of it in an unsterilized patch of skin. The air bubbles are not a huge factor when injecting into fatty tissue, but I was not pleased when I found out later on that I'd taken more interferon than I needed.

SECTION 8

CLINICAL TRIALS: OPTIONS & CHOICES

Keeping an open mind for treatment options

There's a good chance you know by now that treating HCV, either with the two- or three-drug program, isn't a walk in the park. We're dealing with a very serious illness with serious ramifications and its treatment needs equally serious consideration. Admittedly I came to my treatment research with a bias. I'd been into health food and alternative medicine for many years and therefore tended to lean in that direction. The problem with leaning too heavily in one direction or another, whether it be in our health habits or just about anything else in life, is that at some point we may need to change our direction in order to expand our options. Oh yes, the dreaded C-word, *change*; we humans are not overly fond of change. Once we establish a groove we like to settle in and get comfy. Don't ask us to change our diet, or our lifestyle, we are just fine without too much information, thank you very much. However, it doesn't take long for a groove to turn into a rut. As a teacher I once knew said, "The only difference between a rut and a grave is one of depth." HCV can shake up our comfy little world in a hurry. Even though we may not be overly fond of change and rearranging our comfort zone, we still have the option of adaptability to save our skins when called upon to do so.

I have to admit that in the long run my somewhat stubborn bias towards all natural therapies probably hindered me from exploring viable treatment options and being cured years sooner. Natural therapies aided greatly after the initial stage of diagnosis to lower my liver enzymes in record time. My family doctor, who was not overly inclined towards alternative medicines, was very impressed with how fast my enzyme levels dropped and the overall progress I initially made. But I do feel that I would have been better off with a broader approach early on. But as many of us have experienced, it's challenging enough to change but even harder to do so in the face of misleading horror stories and factual scarcity.

Human nature is a funny thing, it often takes a big kick in the pants to get us to shift gears and explore a different direction. Sometimes we just have to be willing to admit that what we're doing may not be the best option for us and start looking for a new approach. A new approach doesn't mean we chuck all our views but simply that we expand them to allow a greater scope of possibilities. A positive open minded attitude can help keep things in balance and not allow our groove to get too deep.

Clinical trials with a difference

I've recently heard of clinical trials for HCV that involve the use of Chinese herbal remedies. It will be interesting to see the conclusions that these trials bring about and their effect on the virus. Whatever benefit there may be will add to the knowledge base of information and may be of assistance for those who do not want to or are prevented from undertaking conventional drug treatment therapy for one reason or another. Any herbs or supplements found to give the liver positive support and help to slow the degenerative process would be a big help for many. HCV treatment is served well with a broad range of considerations. Not everyone is going to come to the same conclusion about their treatment but everyone is entitled to accurate information in order to make that decision.

On the flip side it needs to be mentioned that there is a fairly long list of natural products, including some Chinese herbs that are proven to be harmful and others that are potentially harmful to a challenged liver. I was provided with a lengthy list of harmful or questionable herbs by my treatment doctor. The following (courtesy of hevadvocate.org) is a list of some of the more common herbs and supplements to moderate or avoid; your doctor should be able to provide more thorough information.

- Iron, vitamin A, and vitamin C should be minimized
- Niacin should be taken in only normally recommended amounts

- Black Cohosh
- Blue-green Algae
- Borage
- Chaparral
- Comfrey
- Dong Quai
- Germander
- Jin Bu Huan
- Kava

- Ma-Huang
- Mistletoe
- Pennyroyal
- Sassafras
- Scullcap
- Shark Cartilage
- Valerian
- Yohimbe

To treat now or to wait

In the spring of 2011 a new chapter in HCV treatment was started. The long awaited triple therapy that promised a second chance for the genotype 1 non-responders was available at last. And even for those genotype 1s who had not gone through treatment, the much higher success rate shown in clinical trials made the prospect of treatment much more attractive. Even as the triple therapy was being launched there were a number of advanced clinical trials underway in the U.S. and other countries. Protease inhibitors are a class of drugs referred to as direct acting antivirals. Their function is to primarily slow the reproduction of the virus so the interferon and ribavirin can more effectively deal with the virus. Think of it this way, if an enemy has an almost unlimited capacity to keep new troops in the field it's hard to win the battle. DAAs stop or at least greatly slow down the number of new arrivals. The most advanced clinical trials underway are testing DAAs that are easier to tolerate than the current protease inhibitors. Considering that protease inhibitors are the first major development in over a decade it's fairly amazing to see new developments coming to the fore so rapidly. There are also promising results with therapies that don't include the use of interferon at all. Interferon has been the armor piercing bullet in the fight against HCV from the beginning. Even in its cruder form in the 1990s it did achieve some positive results. Later, when combined with ribavirin in its new pegylated form, it achieved much greater success. The challenge with interferon has always been its side effects. Many of the negative side effects in HCV treatment come from interferon. To replace interferon with something that does not produce its most challenging side effects and also does not require an injection drug would indeed be a major step forward. With the advancement of DAAs there is the hope of paving the way for less intrusive drugs to deliver the knockout blow to eliminating the virus. Another major goal of these efforts is also to shorten the treatment time for achieving a cure, especially for genotype 1. All of this brings a lot of food for thought regarding the timing of potential treatment decisions. It is now summer of 2013 and a friend has just completed taking part in a clinical trial that doesn't use interferon. She is genotype 1 and has failed to respond to two previous attempts at treatment with the two drug therapy, so this is her third attempt at a cure. With a non-interferon program of twenty four weeks she was an early responder and appears to be cured. She still has to wait for the six month post treatment follow up viral load test to claim her victory. Many in the health community, and of course HCV patients, are awaiting the completion of these trials with great hope for the future of HCV treatments.

Standing at the crossroads (an' we ain't singin' the blues)

So, again we stand at a crossroads of treatment decisions. The question of whether to treat now or wait depends on many considerations. The best thing to do is to stay abreast of developing treatment options while monitoring your condition and consulting with your medical providers. Time is a factor in considering treatment options. Fortunately, HCV liver degeneration tends to move slowly. All factors of one's condition, including age and whether cirrhosis is present or not and any other considerations that might affect the decision need to be discussed with a knowledgeable specialist. Clinical trials and approval of new drugs move slowly and that's a good thing in the long run. Some estimate that a new DAA therapy that still includes interferon and ribavirin might be available by the end of 2013 or 2014. The current projection for when an interferon-free treatment option might be available is around 2014 to 2015. And yes, it's still all a best guess at this point. It's fairly safe to say with the progress that is being made towards faster and easier treatment options that HCV treatment will look much different in the years to come.

Stay tuned

As clinical trials move forward the buzz is gaining momentum. How soon will these new drugs be available and even more important in the long run, what will their side effects be? How soon will these new drugs totally eliminate interferon? Will all genotypes benefit from these new treatment options? Lots of questions are swirling around. And I'm sure much information will be making the rounds, some accurate and some not so accurate. Let's stay tuned and make sure we go to good sources for our information. At last there are many sources of good information on the internet through a number of nonprofit HCV advocacy groups as well as from the scientific community. As always, be sure to check your sources.

SECTION 9

PRETREATMENT/ GETTING READY

Conventional treatment cost factors

HCV treatment drugs are not cheap and are not really meant to be purchased by individuals. It's kind of like the old joke, "If you have to ask how much it costs, you probably can't afford it." As a very rough figure, back in 2010 when I was researching treatment costs, I came up with a monthly cost of about $2,000 for interferon and ribavirin and almost that again for doctors and lab fees. For genotype 1s with the new protease inhibitor that cost would be more, much more. If you have insurance it can still be pricey with co-pays and deductibles. The drug companies have programs to help those who have high deductibles and high out-of-pocket expenses. It's to their advantage to have you use their drugs so they are very helpful in making that happen. If you don't have insurance then explore some of the government programs to see if you qualify for any medical aid options. There is a resource section at the end of the book for information on patient assistance with the drug companies as well as government programs. Getting on a list to participate in a clinical trial is another viable option.

Treatment on the cheap

If you don't have medical insurance it is rather easy to get interferon and ribavirin for free. The process generally involves a short phone interview with a rep from the drug company. They mainly want to check your insurance status and that you are under their yearly household income level. Incidentally, the income level maximum is close to twice what a lot of people with decent jobs make, so it's a very easy to qualify. There is some marginal paperwork involved but it is a very straightforward, easy process. You will need to provide information about your treatment doctor as they will be the ones the drug company will complete the process with and send the drugs to. I recently contacted a rep at the drug company that I received my interferon and ribavirin from to inquire about any possible changes brought about with the additional drugs that are now being used. He informed me that the process for patient assistance is still the same and covers all treatment drugs at this time.

Another difficult challenge for the uninsured is figuring how to cover the costs of doctor's visits and lab fees. Weekly or even biweekly office visits and labs can get expensive. A full viral load test is somewhere in the neighborhood of $800. A saving grace may be found in your community in the form of a clinic with a sliding scale for the cost of office and lower lab fees for cash patients. You may need to get creative and do some digging but that's where the determination factor comes in. Often treatment and support are not found in one easy location but in two separate facilities. I went through treatment without medical insurance on a cash basis. My cost averaged out to about $200 per month plus some additional upfront costs for tests and exams prior to treatment. There are programs to assist with lab fees for those with lower incomes or no insurance, or who are self-employed. Truthfully this area of how to pay for treatment, especially the lab and doctor fees, can be a big challenge. Just keep working with your doctor and social services and as mentioned explore the possibility of being part of a clinical trial.

Getting ready to get ready

Some of what is covered in this section on preparation for treatment refers to what needs to be done or is advisable before undertaking conventional drug therapy. Other items deal more with what happens during the actual treatment so you will have a heads up beforehand.

Preparation is half the battle

A crazy thing happened one day at the HCV support group that I attend, and sometimes lead. It was one of those seemingly out of the blue situations that make you wonder what just happened. Afterwards we were all sitting there with our jaws dropped. The incident illustrates the need for preparation rather well.

About ten minutes into our weekly one-hour HCV support group meeting a lady showed up looking slightly bewildered. It was her first time at one of our meetings and she asked, "Is this where the interferon is?" That was a rather strange question so we proceeded to explain that it was an HCV support group and we would be happy to answer any questions she might have about interferon and treatment in general. She took a seat and we explained to her that we were having a discussion about side effects and how some of the folks were doing who were currently going through treatment. Sometimes we just give folks a chance to ask questions if they're new and half scared out of their wits or on treatment and need support with a particular issue.

As the meeting progressed she didn't say much, just sat quietly and only asked one question about a point that came up. Toward the end of the meeting one of the group leaders mentioned treatment prep and that sometimes it could take two or three months and in some cases even longer to get ready for treatment. All of a sudden this lady started to get rather agitated and almost shouted, "Two or three months?" We started to explain that there are necessary checkups for treatment preparation and to insure that it's a safe and viable option for patients. But we didn't get very far. She stood up gathering her things and blurted out, "I thought I would get my shot at the end of this meeting!" That's when our jaws just dropped and we realized the significance of her initial question "Is this where the interferon is?" We really wanted to help her and find out how in the world she'd been led to think you can just show up and start treatment but unfortunately she was in such a state that all she could say was "I've been told I need to start treatment NOW," and with that she stormed out. We could only hope she'd come back because she either seriously misunderstood something her doctor told her or just got some crazy information. The poor lady did not have a clue as to the commitment involved in starting treatment. As we already covered, commitment is a key element, and now we add preparation. Of course education and knowledge are an ongoing aspect of the process as well. You don't just show up like you're getting a flu shot, you've got to be educated, prepared, and checked out.

The preparation for my first treatment was fairly minimal which led to me having a challenging time. For the second attempt I was much more prepared having attended group for almost three months beforehand. All the prep and information allowed me to better manage my side effects as well as minimize their severity. For example, just being informed about how vital it is to drink adequate amounts of water made a big difference. I also went into my second treatment feeling ready and supported, which was a real boost to start off on a positive note.

Why all the fuss anyway?

There are two basic reasons for the pretreatment checkups. One is to determine a person's present level of health or lack thereof as the case may be. Preexisting conditions such as diabetes or any number of serious illnesses need to be taken into consideration to evaluate if a person is healthy enough for the stress of treatment and if there might be any complications with existing medications. Sometimes a patient will need to get an existing condition under better control or more stable before starting another treatment program. That is what we wanted to share with Ms. "Give-it-to-me-now." These are all common-sense precautions. The checkups also serve to establish a baseline in case anything comes up. For instance, as we covered in the section on testing, your doctor will want to know what your blood factors look like so when you start treatment he/she can tell the extent of the drug's effects on red and white blood cells and platelets as you progress through the treatment.

Common pretreatment tests and procedures

There may be specific tests ordered to cover existing conditions, but apart from that here is a list of the basic tests and procedures that are commonly ordered and the reasons for them.

- A complete physical will be done to check your overall health.

- If you haven't had one recently, an ultrasound exam will be done to look at your liver and other organs. Ultrasound can help determine if there is any swelling or abnormalities present. It is often used as a preliminary exam to determine if further testing/exams are necessary.

- Depending on findings from the ultrasound and other factors including age and how long one has possibly had the virus, a liver biopsy* might be ordered. A biopsy will show if there is any fibrosis or cirrhosis (degrees of tissue damage and scarring) present in the liver.

- A complete vision test with retinal scan will be ordered. Vision can shift around, it is strange, but it does happen to some. Interesting that in Chinese medicine the eyes are directly linked to the liver. I didn't notice any vision change during my first treatment. But during my second go, I had my only optical migraine ever, and the prescription for my glasses shifted, and then went back after treatment.

- Time to visit the dentist. This is important because we don't want any dental challenges like an abscess cropping up leading to a serious infection. With lowered white blood cell counts an infection of this sort could become serious very fast. We had a lady in treatment end up in the hospital from a tooth abscess. Under normal conditions she would have gone to the dentist and gotten antibiotics and that would have been it. But with her lowered white blood cell count due to treatment, her body wasn't able to hold the infection at bay. She had to wait over the weekend to see the dentist and by then the infection had spread and she was in serious trouble. The more prepared and healthier we are prior to treatment the better.

*I know, yikes, a biopsy. Let's cover what a biopsy is all about to alleviate any panic. When I was preparing for my first treatment my doctor told me I should get a biopsy. Up until he explained the procedure I had been under the impression it was a major deal. I thought I would be cut open and a chunk of my liver would be extracted. Actually it only involves a special long, fairly thin hollow needle that is inserted into the liver to extract a very small segment of liver material. This sample of tissue is then carefully examined under a microscope to determine any damage that the liver might have sustained from the presence of the virus. There is a lot of prep and a number of people involved but the actual insertion and extraction of the needle only takes a few seconds to complete. A local anesthetic is used and most of the time you don't feel much of anything. My biopsy and that of many people I have spoken with were not a major deal and the information that results from it is of vital importance. If I would have known earlier what the actual procedure for a liver biopsy was I would have had one done years earlier. There are a small percentage of people who've had complications from a needle biopsy ranging from mild to severe. As with most things of this nature, talk to your doctor and get informed.

Stages of liver disease

Now that we know a liver biopsy is not as challenging a procedure as we might have imagined, we need to understand what purpose it serves and why we might need one in the first place. Over time as the liver fights against the invasion of HCV virus, it progressively becomes more affected by the long term effects of the battle. Not everyone has the same degree of liver damage but the potential is there and a biopsy helps to determine the level of liver damage that has occurred up to that point.

Sometimes it's difficult to understand what all this business of virus invasion and potential liver damage is all about and what exactly is going on inside of the body. Let's look at the process of liver damage in simple terms without a lot of medical jargon. Once the HCV virus enters the body through the blood stream, it is carried to the liver as a natural function of the liver filtering the blood. Upon entering the liver the virus finds that it has all the components it needs to set up shop. The virus, which is very small, enters a liver cell and uses its resources to create more virus cells to release back into the blood stream to be carried to other parts of the liver. Simply put, the liver, with all of its many functions, is the perfect environment the virus needs to set up its own little HCV production facility. The liver becomes a HCV virus factory churning out trillions of new HCV virions (individual virus cells) on a daily basis.

Left alone the virus just does what everything else on earth does, makes more of itself to insure the survival of its kind. Unfortunately for us our liver is its food source. Our immune system recognizes the invader and goes into action. In response to this foreign invasion our immune system sends in its own immune cell warriors to battle the virus. And if our immune system is strong it can knock out the virus and be done with it before it becomes chronic. Close to 25% of folks who are infected can fight it on their own and they're done. But for the rest of us, the counter attack goes on much longer. In fact it goes on from day one for as long as we and the virus are together.

What's going on in there anyway?

This is what the battle scene looks like. Our immune response targets and attacks the cells that the virus has invaded. As the cells are being nuked by our immune system, they are damaged, and when the body rebuilds these damaged cells it results in what is essentially scar tissue. The unfortunate problem is that these attacks do not have the necessary fire power to kill the virus itself, so they only serve to damage liver cells. The longer the battle rages the more scarring occurs. This battle scene has been going on for year after year in our liver, no days off, 24/7! As the fight continues the damaged liver cells increase to the point of scarred cells joining together forming what is called fibrosis. Scar tissue is linked to other scar tissue and a string-like fiber is created. As the scarring increases the fibrosis spreads (bridges) creating larger areas of non-functioning liver cells. Liver damage is defined by the degree or amount of scarring that has occurred. In its final stage, fibrosis becomes so extensive that the scar tissue has replaced a substantial portion of the liver's healthy cells. At the point that fibrosis encircles large areas of the liver producing nodules of dead cells and the liver becomes harder and shrunken, we have what is called cirrhosis. I know, not a pretty picture, and not everyone gets to that stage but many do over an extended period of time.

Progression to cirrhosis is determined to some extent by how long one has had the virus and also how old we are. The liver tends to experience faster deterioration as we age. The old school of thought was, let's see how things go, the degeneration moves slowly. As more data is accumulated that perspective is starting to shift towards doing treatment sooner than later since the younger we are the more responsive we are to treatment. Also with earlier treatment the prospect of developing cirrhosis is virtually eliminated if it isn't already present. Additionally, since it's usually many years after the onset of HCV before its diagnoses, most people will often have some level of fibrosis, and possibly even cirrhosis by that time. From the study of liver disease and its progression, the medical community has identified four stages of degeneration.

Stages of Degeneration:
Stage One: Mild/beginning fibrosis
Stage Two: Moderate fibrosis
Stage Three: Severe fibrosis
Stage Four: Cirrhosis

Vertex Pharmaceuticals states in one of their HCV brochures that according to a study conducted in 2008 approximately 41% of those who have had HCV for at least thirty years have cirrhosis. That statistic presents a strong motivation for thorough testing and identifying the extent of liver damage. Once that is known you and your doctor can best determine your course of action. The fact that cirrhosis was detected in my biopsy was a determining factor in my decision to get treated sooner rather than later.

Getting ready, getting healthy

Having HCV is a challenge to the liver and to our overall health. The healthier we can be in spite of that, the better we will handle treatment whether it's conventional drug therapy or an alternative treatment. HCV is not an excuse to have bad health habits; it's a reason to have good ones.

It's a really good idea to start anything that will be beneficial to your treatment program before treatment actually begins. Mild exercise like walking is a good practice during treatment even when you don't feel like it. It gets your lymph system moving and helps shake off some of the malaise. It's a fairly easy way to get some activity instead of just sitting around thinking about how crappy you feel. But if you haven't developed a walking habit before treatment, it's going to be hard to get in the groove after you start. The same holds true with most of the following suggestions, they are all good for you anyway.

One more lap around the living room

At times any form of extra effort might not be what you have in mind. A lot of how we feel comes from our heads. We often don't "feel" like doing anything because we're feeling ill and down. Sometimes it helps to just mentally "park" your head, put your shoes on and get out the door. You may only walk to the mailbox or a block down the road and back, but that's okay. It's as much about getting out of your head as getting out of the door. We're not talking about a heavy-duty program, just something to move you off the couch and get some fresh air. It can be anything, even a stroll in the back yard or a few bounces on a rebounder. If you have any kind of movement program that you enjoy like Yoga, T'ai Chi, Pilates, or something of that nature, those are all good for moving the body. Having a pre-established routine is a plus and of course you can modify your activity to meet your current energy level. Again it's much easier to continue an established momentum than starting one after beginning treatment.

Water, the holy elixir of HCV treatment

If you were to ask anyone in the support group I attended what they considered the one most important thing to do during treatment, I'm sure they would all say DRINK YOUR WATER! No kidding, the importance of drinking adequate amounts of water (preferably bottled or filtered, not tap water unless you have your own well and it's not chlorinated) cannot be overstated. Drinking plenty of water does a number of good things for you in general and is especially important during treatment. The meds tend to dehydrate the body and also produce a lot of toxins. While water is rehydrating the body, in the process it also helps flush out toxins. We know the liver filters toxins from the body so drinking plenty of water helps lessen that load on the liver. When you don't drink enough water during treatment there is a much greater chance of having headaches and feeling more fatigued and experiencing greater side effects in general. Almost everyone in the support group who neglected their water intake even for a day saw the difference. It is also important to maintain the water regime after treatment has ended since it can take several months to get the drugs out of your system.

Personal water testimony

My first treatment did not stress the importance of drinking water. Even though my first treatment only lasted twelve weeks, the side effects were worse and I believe that water made a big difference during my second treatment. One thing that can happen during treatment is brain fog, forgetfulness, short term memory challenges, and it's even worse than normal for us older guys. During my first treatment I worked in a bank where I used a number of software applications to record information going from one screen to another to complete a transaction. By the second month of treatment my short term memory started having some serious challenges. During the data entry process when I would shift screens, as soon as a new screen came up I totally forget what I was doing. I didn't have a clue as to what the next step was and what I was supposed to do. I had to stare at the screen for a moment until my brain kicked back in and remembered the next step in the sequence so that I could activate the next command. This happened on a regular basis for over a month. An automatic process that I'd carried out for a number of years just vanished in an instant. It slowly got better after stopping treatment. Even though the shifting-screen-brain-function problem got better I still had other short term memory challenges for several months after stopping treatment. The interesting thing is that during my second treatment, which lasted twice as long as the first, and where I drank plenty of water, I didn't experience anywhere near the same level of memory challenge. Sure, sometimes I'd forget what I was talking about in mid-sentence but not too frequently and nothing as severe as my first experience.

The water formula

Water intake is individually tailored for each person based on their weight using a set formula. You can drink more but you must drink at least the minimum derived from the formula. Divide your body weight by two. Half your body weight in ounces is the amount of water you need to drink every day. Say for example you weigh one hundred and sixty pounds, half of that would be eighty. So eighty ounces would be the magic number. Since there are thirty-two ounces in a quart, eighty ounces would equal two and a half quarts of water. Round any odd number up to the nearest half quart to keep things simple and drink that amount each day without fail. The more you weigh the more water you'll need. Interestingly enough, two quarts equals those eight glasses of water that we've heard forever that we should drink each day. So here is another case of HCV helping us do what we should be doing anyway. Drinking more is fine but don't go crazy and overdo your water intake. There can be problems with massive water intake. Stay close to the formula and everything will be fine. My daily allotment was just over two quarts and some days I'd drink three. Four wouldn't have hurt me; I just would have never left the bathroom! Also if you drink too much you'll flush out healthy minerals that your body needs.

What water is and is not

Water is not caffeinated tea, coffee, soda, or anything with sugar added. If you want to add fresh lemon juice or something of that nature because drinking water is a challenge (I've heard people say this) that's fine. Even mild unsweetened herb tea is okay. Once again, try to avoid drinking tap water. Even if you've gotten used to the taste of chlorine and other nasty things that are now considered normal in our tap water, your liver doesn't need the extra work of filtering those things out of your body. Especially not at the now increased volume you'll be taking in. One thing to consider for treatment and into your healthier future, is investing in a water filter that hooks up to your kitchen tap. At the very least you can get a pitcher water filter like those from Pur or Britta. The tap-attached filters are cheaper in the long run but whatever works for your budget and can get you going is fine. Buying those cases of bottled water can get pricey and produces a ton of extra plastic for disposal. That said, having some of those on hand for quick grab and go may be helpful at times. To be clear, if you only have or decide that tap water is what you want to drink then go ahead and do that. It's better to drink that than not take in adequate water.

Keeping track of water intake

I used a thirty-two ounce water bottle that is made of heavy-duty plastic (glass or stainless steel is really the better way to go). If you have one of those old aluminum one quart canteens from your Boy/Girl Scout days, please throw it away. Aluminum leaches into food and water and is quite toxic. Cooking with straight aluminum that doesn't have a stainless steel coating or other not toxic coating is not a good idea either. I drank a little over two bottles a day, sometimes three, and there were times I'd forget whether I was filling bottle number two or three, due to the foggy brain thing. I ended up getting a couple extra bottle tops and numbered them and switched them out with each refill. Some folks just get as many quart bottles (or half quart/16 oz.) as they need each day and don't have to worry about numbering. Every morning you just faithfully set out your day's supply and never leave home without a bottle or two. You're maybe thinking it's weird that you would even need a system for keeping track of a few bottles of water. Trust me; it's not weird at all, just a way to help that foggy brain during treatment. Do not think that you can mentally keep track of how much water you drink without a system that actually measures the amount. Under the best of circumstances it's really hard to drink enough water by just wanting to. I'm going to be blunt; you will probably suffer if you try that. It's not a bad idea to clean your water bottle out every once in a while to avoid the possibility of mold. Fill the bottle with hot water and a little bleach, let it sit for an hour or so and then wash and rinse out really well.

Sleep/Rest/De-stress

Sleep is essential for your body to replenish the day's spent energy (especially when you don't have a lot to start with) and repair and restore vital organ systems which obviously include the liver. One problem that tends to come up is that the treatment drugs can disrupt sleep cycles making a good night's sleep a challenge. Further, adding to the problem is the amount of water you're drinking during treatment. Getting up to go to the bathroom several times at night doesn't help the situation. I always put my water intake as a priority so if I didn't get it all in before bed, well that was too bad for me. That said, it's a good idea at least in theory to get your daily water allotment in a few hours before bed time.

So this is what menopause is like

Every post-menopausal woman I've ever spoken with about my night sweats said something like "Yeah, now you know a little of what menopause is like!" Often I'd go through anywhere from three to six t-shirt changes a night. I was getting up to use the bathroom anyway, so I got the most out of my wake-ups. I set up one of those folding wooden clothes racks and kept a supply of t-shirts and bath towels handy. Using bath towels was easier than changing sheets all the time. If you find your sleep disrupted a lot and you're in a relationship, it may be best for both of you to sleep separately during parts of treatment. No sense everyone getting poor sleep and adding to the stress and cranky level of the household.

HCV on the job

If you're planning on continuing to work during treatment be sure to let your immediate supervisor and those you work closely with know that you might need to take longer rest breaks than usual. Don't try to tough it out and not tell the people you work with. You don't always need to give a lot of details, just say you're dealing with some medical issues if that's more comfortable than talking to them about your possibly wild and reckless youth. During my first treatment if I hit the wall I'd just go out to my car and take a short nap in the parking lot. I parked at the back of the lot. I told folks I might need to do that and it just made it easier because when I really needed to I could just check out without stressing about it. It sure is easier to take a ten to twenty minute nap than pretend to work when you're totally zonked out and no good to anyone anyway.

Depending on your job situation you may want to consider working part time if at all possible. It might come down to that anyway so you might as well give it some thought early on. If you can work it out to take an extended leave, that might not be a bad idea either. One person I know who is a heavy equipment operator (like major earth moving stuff) decided that he didn't want to risk running that kind of equipment if he wasn't feeling too great, a wise move on his part. He also knew that construction guys aren't all that warm and fuzzy towards each other at times and that treatment can make you a little edgy and downright cranky. He didn't want to be in a situation that was ripe for confrontation without his usual good natured defenses in place, another wise move.

Stress 101

If you have HCV you're already stressed whether you know it or not. Hepatitis by definition equals a stressed liver which in turn adds stress to other organs and their related functions. We might not even be aware of these stresses on a conscious level but they are there nonetheless. That's just the way the body works, it's not something we can control. Knowing this can give us a big heads up to realize that all of these stresses, plus the addition of the treatment drugs, can easily add up to some challenges that we need to prepare for. Even though each of us handles stress in our own way, there are some factors that apply to all of us. It's common knowledge that things like adequate sleep, good nutrition, exercise, rest, and a host of other factors can minimize our stress levels. While we want to pay attention to maintaining those healthy habits, we also realize that treatment can knock a lot of those factors for a loop. In the face of uncertain stress potential, one of our most valuable coping tools is awareness. Our awareness that unusual stressors may crop up can help us tremendously. The challenge, of course, is to maintain that awareness in the face of changing conditions. It can be hard to be aware of something that we haven't experienced before because we simply don't know what to look for. Besides the "watch out for weird stuff" heads up, which by the way, will come in handier than we might think, this is where our support system comes into play. A gentle reminder about our stress levels and how we are coping can be very helpful for keeping things in balance. The important thing for us to remember is to be open and grateful for the help and not become reactive or defensive. A few "be aware and listen" Post-its on the bathroom mirror and elsewhere may not be a bad idea.

Here is a major awareness tip, stress is rarely caused by others or situations outside of ourselves. That's right, blaming others because we are stressed is just shifting the blame. We need to just own up to the fact that we are stressed and look for healthy ways to deal with *our* stress. The exercise section also applies to helping with stress as a means of coping. One guy in our support group discovered that hot baths and hot tubs were just the thing he needed when he was feeling stressed or just funky from treatment. Incidentally this is the same guy who ran heavy equipment. I just have to give him points for facing situations with a calm realistic approach; we can all learn something from that.

At some point a "New Normal" will come in handy

The "new normal" concept came up during a support group meeting that was being led by a mental health worker at the clinic where some of us received our treatment. One fellow we'll call Jason was having a tough time during treatment, but not because of any of the usual side effects. Every week he came to group and proclaimed that he felt miserable. He actually looked much better than some of us going through treatment and he didn't have that many side effects except a bit of fatigue. His main complaint was that he wasn't getting to the gym as regular as before and he was having trouble maintaining his well-toned body!

Before starting treatment Jason spent a lot of time in the gym and it was a large part of his life and routine. He couldn't do that as regularly now and that was messing with his head. The mental health worker patiently tried to explain that part of his anxiety was from trying to hold onto and maintain his life exactly like it was before he started treatment, his "old normal." He couldn't see that he was putting an unrealistic demand on himself under his current circumstances. Instead of being grateful that his new normal allowed him to get to the gym three times a week, instead of six, he just saw the glass half empty and that was a miserable situation for him. If you know you tend to be part of the glass half empty crowd, I would gently recommend that you really try to pay attention to that tendency so it doesn't make challenging situations worse.

Jason's situation also serves as a good example of how treatment can differ from one individual to another and the difference that attitude can make. While some of us were trying to get out the door for a ten minute walk, another guy is doing weight training three days a week. If I got out for a short walk I was happy, if I didn't, well, there was always tomorrow. We really have to be kind to ourselves and not stress over unrealistic expectations and demands. And sometimes we just need to hang in there with the old this-too-shall-pass to deal with what comes up. Even though treatment can sometimes feel like it will last forever it's good to remember that all our favorite activities will still be there for us after we're done.

Establishing your support system; group and personal

My first twelve week treatment was undertaken without a support group combined with very little knowledge of what to expect. Because I didn't have the necessary information it also meant that those close to me didn't have any real information to fall back on either. They had no support for their own understanding or peace of mind. Unfortunately, instead of offering support they often unknowingly added to the overall stress. They were not able to provide gentle reminders to help me when necessary and we all had a pretty tough time. Being a significant person to someone going through treatment, whether as a spouse, family member, or close friend, can be very challenging. It's important for your loved ones and personal support group to be as informed as you are about various aspects of treatment. At some point you will probably need to rely on them to help you get a balanced perspective on things. Healing HCV is rarely a solo journey and with its challenging and at times unpredictable nature, we can use some level-headed support. Having a support group consisting of people going through treatment as well as at least one person who has completed treatment can be of immeasurable help. We also open our group to people exploring treatment options which allows for a good exchange of ideas and information. While I was going through treatment myself I found that helping and encouraging others about their treatment options not only helped them but also made me feel that my challenges and treatment experiences were more worthwhile. It helped to focus on encouraging and supporting others as opposed to just fixating on myself.

Riding the emotional roller coaster

There were times during my first treatment when I didn't realize my emotional state was out of balance and my perspective on situations was distorted. A big part of being human is the challenge of keeping a clear head and not letting our emotions run away with us. That challenge becomes more acute when on treatment. As was mentioned, awareness of the potential for emotional imbalance is a big heads up for ourselves and those close to us. It's the first step towards keeping things from getting out of hand. We may think that we're going to be the exception to the rule and can keep our emotional stuff from getting "that bad." It doesn't have to get that bad, it just has to get a little off balance to challenge our normal coping mechanisms. When we don't have the clarity or knowledge to understand what is happening, it can lead to a lot of confusion and frustration, which in turn can make challenging emotional situations much worse than they need be.

The second time I underwent treatment I was much calmer and more balanced. There were still some emotional roller coaster rides, but I was better able to work through them without dragging others into the drama. In part my earlier experience gave me some insights to guide me but mainly I feel that having support and education made the biggest difference. That may be why I'm such a big advocate of treatment support groups for HCV sufferers at all stages of their journey. I can attest to the difference it makes to have support and reliable information versus struggling on one's own; it's a world of difference.

During treatment you may not feel like hanging out with friends and family very much. When we don't feel too great we're often not very sociable. It can be a great comfort to have a support group where you can just share how you feel without a lot of extra explanations. If you don't have an available group it's good to have at least one person who you can count on to lend an ear and provide support when you need it or are feeling low. If you can establish contact, even long distance, with someone who's gone through treatment, so much the better. In any case, let those close to you know that you may not be very sociable during treatment. Let them also know that you appreciate their support and that you do want to keep in touch at least by phone, e-mail, or text if not in person. Make sure they understand it's the treatment and not a personal thing if you aren't up to your normal social activities. For some, all of this may not be a large issue, I just know for me it was. I had a lot of stuff going on emotionally and at times my life felt like one big soap opera. And that was before starting treatment!

Maintaining spiritual & emotional well being

Getting in touch with that which feeds and sustains us spiritually and emotionally prior to beginning treatment is a good idea. For some of us this is a daily practice and for others maybe not so much. But for all of us once we start treatment we can use all the help we can get from whatever levels we can connect with. Even if you have a fair number of side effects and treatment is kicking your butt it will be your attitude, faith, and grit, or combination thereof, that will make the biggest difference for you; along with that support system we talked about.

The nasty F-word . . . Fatigue

It is worth noting that the most prevalent common challenge that people with HCV have is some level of fatigue. Here I am addressing fatigue not as a side effect of treatment, but merely as a result of having the virus. For many who have carried the virus long term, fatigue can become a major issue in their lives.

The inability to work and earn a living is a humbling experience, but not all that uncommon among HCV sufferers. I've met a number of people with advanced stages of HCV who have had financial challenges mainly due to how fatigue limited their employment opportunities. It's unsettling and a real shock to find that all of a sudden the ability to work full time or even part time is no longer an option. The possibility of fatigue affecting one's ability to function in the workplace does need to be kept in mind.

The severity of fatigue can vary from almost none to severe. Fatigue, if it occurs, can be slow or swift in its development. For some this will not be an issue, for others it's something to keep an eye on. And for those who have ongoing fatigue I hope you can take a little comfort in knowing others have dealt with similar issues and lived to tell the tale.

It can be challenging to not allow our weakened state to define who we are. No doubt about it, it can be depressing, and depression can make us feel like we are lesser beings because we just don't have the energy level to function like our friends, family, and coworkers (providing we still have coworkers). It can be frustrating on many levels. You look fairly okay, but there are days that you can hardly move your body around. A friend who had hep C for a long time once said that moving is body was like driving his first car, a beater '54 Buick with a number of bad cylinders. Slow, awkward, and at times embarrassing.

After all was said and done, it was the issue with fatigue that drove me to move a few mountains and get treated. And for me, it was worth it.

Digging deep and holding tight

Some days in the midst of all the challenges of getting ready for and then later when going through treatment, I just had to let go of all the head stuff that stress can bring up and say okay this is what I need to do and focus on dealing with that one thing, one step at a time. Adopting a "one step at a time" attitude during HCV treatment can come in handy. Before I started my treatment I met a fellow who went through treatment in the '90s. There was no ribavirin or pegylated interferon available back then, just the original interferon that required three to four shots a week. He did that treatment for two full years before he cleared the virus. How he did that and also managed to come out with his marriage intact is beyond me. He gets credit for sticking with the treatment and his wife gets credit for putting up with him doing it. No small thing for either of them. That gave me some serious perspective whenever I'd hit a hard spot.

I believe that everything we experience has the opportunity to be a blessing if we dig deep enough to find it. There's nothing like getting stripped down to the bare essentials of keeping body and soul together to give us a larger perspective on life. We may even experience a sense of gratitude for life's more basic blessings and the people we share our life with. As an old Montana cowboy I knew used to say: "Having a roof over your head, beans on the table, and a partner or good friend, are never to be taken for granted." At some point you just have to gear up, get things in place as best you can, and go for it. The more knowledge, support, spiritual sustenance, and positive attitude you can muster the better. Some will have a harder time with symptoms and/or treatment than others. And then there's the guy in our support group who has a headache, one time, during his yearlong treatment. Go figure!

Giving credit where credit is due

Not everyone who has HCV was a drug addict or spent time in jail. Not everyone, but a large percentage of HCV sufferers were infected by IV drug use and/or jail house tattoos. I'll tell the truth, my first support group meeting was a shocker. I'd been a middle class kid who got swept up in the drug culture like a lot of others at that time. Yeah, I pushed the envelope a bit farther than most of my friends and got into the hard stuff but that ended by age twenty-four. By then I'd spent a year in jail, two different times, for possession of small amounts of drugs and large quantities of stupid. But I was still a kid and got myself sorted out and on the straight and narrow. Not so with a good number of the people I was sitting next to and across the table from in my support group. A lot of these folks had traveled a hard road for a long time and it was very apparent. Some were still trying to get clean from drugs or alcohol in order to start treatment. As we introduced ourselves and shared a little about our situation I heard myself saying I'd been drug free for close to forty years. It was somewhat surreal in a sense to see my former self reflected in the people around me. It was one of those there-but-for-the-grace-of-God-go-I moments. So this is my opportunity to speak to you who have traveled that long challenging road. By this point you've faced a lot of crap in your life and now maybe you're getting ready to start treatment. I just hope you realize that by the time you've kicked whatever habit you had and stopped whatever activities landed you in jail, you've faced more challenges than most people could imagine. Yes, those were self-inflicted situations to a large degree but it didn't make them any easier to conquer, maybe even harder. So please know, there are people who admire your courage and understand where you've been. Take that courage and determination into your treatment and it will serve you well.

Section 10

Going through Treatment

Perspective on side effects

When you stop to think about it there are not that many diseases having a cure procedure as well defined as HCV. Take cancer for example, it doesn't have a set treatment time and hardly ever a reliable cure prognosis. AIDS sufferers have drugs to diminish and in some cases stabilize the effects of the disease, but to date there is no cure for clearing the virus. Those are a couple of hard gigs and of course there are many others. It's important for us not to get so focused on our condition that we lose sight of the fact that many others have equal and maybe even harder challenges. There are many other illnesses that are lifelong incurable conditions that put great stress on the lives of those who are afflicted and their loved ones. So let's keep in mind as we review the upcoming list of side effects that there are other disease treatment programs that have side effects that are at least as challenging as HCV, and some are worse with a far lower probability of an actual cure. The somewhat strange thing about our condition is that it often doesn't affect us as noticeably as many other diseases until the later stages. We often see HCV more as an inconvenience than as the deadly disease it really is. Maybe that's one of the reasons it doesn't get as much attention as it should. It's a slow burn so we're essentially walking time bombs that just haven't gone off yet. I believe keeping things in perspective and having gratitude for the healing potential available can make our journey a bit more tolerable.

One size does not fit all

Before we explore the possible side effects, you might encounter we need to be very clear about one major point: These are *possible* side effects and are not written in stone. As previously mentioned everyone gets their own personalized version of treatment reactions. After all, not everyone reacts to the virus itself in the same way. Some people have relatively few side effects and manage fairly well, while others have a downright challenging time. As we explore the possibilities I will share my own experiences and tips for coping with what came up for me and others in my support group.

The poster child

Since I'll be sharing my personal experiences in regards to each side effect please keep the following in mind as we review the list. I'm a small guy with a light frame; 5'7" tall with normal weight of about 140 lbs. I've had a healthy lifestyle with good diet for a very long time (probably what saved me from total liver failure). Also, I'm extremely sensitive to what I ingest, especially when it comes to prescription drugs. I very rarely take them because unless I absolutely have to, the side effects are often worse than what is ailing me. Besides, except for having HCV, I rarely get sick. I'm telling you this because interferon and ribavirin totally kicked my butt. I was a poster child for side effects and fared much worse than anyone I was going through treatment with.

Treatment was very challenging for me. It was very fortunate for me that I had the genotype 2 short version of treatment.

Not the time to start a family

Special Note: This is a big deal; actually it's a huge deal. Ribavirin has been shown to cause serious birth defects. Women who are of child bearing age will need to obtain a negative pregnancy test immediately before starting treatment and make sure they do not become pregnant during and for six months after treatment. The manufacturer of ribavirin recommends the use of at least two reliable forms of effective contraception during treatment and extending to six months following the completion of treatment. The possibility for birth defects can also be passed on by a male who is on treatment to his partner whether she is on treatment or not. Therefore, a woman who is of child bearing age and sexually active with a male who is on treatment needs to follow the same guidelines during his treatment and for six months after as mentioned above. The treatment kit provided by the pharmaceutical company that furnished the interferon and ribavirin for my treatment actually included a home pregnancy tester.

Side Effects: variations on a theme

I'm going to state this as concisely as possible so that we are all clear on side effects before getting into the laundry list of possibilities.

- The side effects you experience will be dependent on a variety of individual factors.

- Some people get some things and others get others and we often don't know why, so we just have to find ways to deal with it (weekly doctor visits, group support, your own network, and faith keep the wheels rolling).

- No one gets all of them (thank goodness).

- Most everyone gets some of them.

- Some get hardly any.

- And a very rare few get none at all.

- The side effects can be mild, moderate, or severe. They are not to be taken lightly and can be put into proper balance and perspective with your doctor's assistance. Communicate with your doctor; don't hold back any information. Anything that is out of the ordinary and catches your attention is worth bringing to your doctor's attention. It might not appear to be a big deal but then again it might be something that is important for your doctor to keep an eye on or order a test for.

One last thing

If you've gotten your information from individuals or those on the internet who delight in spreading scare stories about HCV treatment with little factual basis, please try to set that aside while we explore the realities of conventional HCV treatment. I know there have been some extremely negative reactions to the treatment drugs and possibly in rare instances even fatal. Unfortunately much of that type of information on the internet is driven more by excess emotion than by solid facts. We ultimately don't know what the realities of many of those situations were and what possible factors were involved because the point is usually not to educate but to induce fear. A good example of this type of fear mongering came from a guy in our support group who told us about a friend of his. His buddy went on treatment for a month, declared it too hard and then went back to injecting street drugs. And now that his friend is an expert on HCV treatment he's doing his best to justify his actions by declaring to all his drug buddies that treatment is a waste of time for healing HCV. If we follow that type of logic what are we to deduce from his actions, that shooting drugs is a better way to go? I'm not trying to minimize actual situations but just saying that spreading fear serves no one. I learned the hard way that a decision based on fear is never a good decision.

The laundry list of possible side effects followed by my experience and tips

Generally speaking the side effects are often at their worst during the first two months of treatment because it takes a while for the body to adjust to these powerful drugs.

Flu-like symptoms: feeling tired and run down, possibly some muscle aches and joint pain, feverish, and possible headaches. Take a couple of ibuprofen (generic Advil) or acetaminophen (generic Tylenol) or something of that nature (check with your doctor).

- If possible, take your shot an hour or so before bedtime along with some basic non-narcotic pain meds as mentioned above. The idea is to sleep through the worst of it.

- Forget normal bedtime, go to bed as early as you need (don't stay up late, that will mess with your sleep cycle, which may get challenging anyway).

Dry skin and rash: this is a pretty common side effect that almost everyone gets to one degree or another.

- The lady from the pharmaceutical company suggested Sarna anti-itch lotion (or generic) mixed with a little olive oil.

- I had a pretty serious rash consisting of large blotches along my spine that drove me a little crazy at times. It lasted for about four months and didn't go away for over a month after treatment was over. Very annoying. Everyone else in the group only had dry skin . . . sheesh!

- I also used some prescription cream, it helped a little.

- In some cases the rash can be severe, let your doctor know what's going on.

Special note regarding Incivek: Both doctors and patients involved in administering or undergoing the triple therapy using Incivek need to be aware of the recent inclusion of a "black box" warning on the drug label. Continuing treatment when a sever rash develops (covering 50% of the body or more) can be life threatening. As stated in an article in the Boston Globe, 12/20/2012: A patient advocate said the enhanced warning is important but shouldn't discourage HCV patients. "Obviously, any time you hear something scary like that, it concerns patients," said Lorren Sandt, Executive Director of Caring Ambassadors, an Oregon nonprofit that supports patients with HCV and other chronic diseases. "But this is a known side effect, and the action that needs to be taken is also known. This shouldn't be a reason for people not to go on therapy if they need to."

Dry tickling cough: I'm told about 25% of folks get this. Usually lasts about six weeks or so. I had a dry cough and couldn't take a deep breath for over four months, a real nuisance.

- Do the basic, drink water, cough drops, cough syrup if it gets bad.

- Your doctor should monitor your lungs during your visits to make sure there isn't anything going on at a deeper level.

Fatigue at many and various levels: We've covered the possible ramifications of fatigue prior to treatment. Now the possible turns into the probable since this is one of the biggest complaints people talk about after starting treatment. Basically it comes down to feeling tired and physically weak and you just don't feel like doing anything.

- Sometimes you just go with that, and sometimes you drag your sorry self off the couch, go for a walk anyway, and try to shake it off.

- Feeling this tired can wear on you after a while and it's important to watch yourself and talk with people, especially your doctor, to make sure it doesn't turn into depression.

- Sometimes the fatigue can be quite severe. I stayed really close to home during treatment except on Fridays when I would drive into the city for my weekly check-up, blood draw, and support group. Friday was also my shopping and take-care-of-business-in-town day. I quickly learned to do the most important errands first. If I had four stops planned I sometimes could only do two before I was just too tuckered out to do the rest. I really had to meter my energy expenditure because there just wasn't much there at times. Again the first couple of months were the hardest. A couple times I barely made it through the grocery checkout line. I was almost to the point of sitting on the floor.

- It's important to not put extra stress and pressure on yourself. We don't want to roll over into the fetal position but we also need to realize that during treatment we have one main job to do, and that is simply to get through treatment. It's a big deal, I will kid you not. You may have no, little, or big side effects, but whatever it is, that's your job, just to get through it. The good news is there is a set end time. It crawls like a snail at times but it does end.

Brain Fog: I already mentioned my going blank between shifting PC screens from my first treatment experience and I do believe that drinking more water made a big difference in alleviating the "fog" during my second treatment.

- I carry my memory in a handy binder called a day planner. I've used a planner for over twenty years. For more years than I care to say, I've had to write down anything that was of any importance and needed to get done or remembered. That practice was extremely useful during treatment.

- A healthy sense of humor can make a big difference. Sometimes we just need to laugh at our plight and not take ourselves too seriously. A lot of these weird annoying side effects are just out of our control and will pass when we're done with treatment.

- At times concentration was a challenge, even more so than normal, and with somewhat of an edge to it. Trying to follow long drawn out conversations on a topic that needed a good deal of focus, like someone sharing a movie plot for example, could be surprisingly difficult and quite tiring. Paying attention in general, especially when it involved a lot of detail, would really stretch my energy and patience.

Even watching a movie could be taxing at times. Every day things that we don't normally pay much attention to can be challenging and possibly carry some additional irritation.

Digestive problems & special diet notes:

- Ribavirin can be hard on the stomach. My biggest challenge was its tendency to adversely affect my already sensitive digestion system. My stomach felt queasy and I had no appetite. Because it's recommended that ribavirin be taken with a meal, I found myself in a real Catch 22. The first time I underwent treatment I didn't handle the ribavirin well and my digestion shut down and made me feel like crap. So the doctor cut my dose in half. The second time around I was informed ahead of time that there is a good reason the doses are what they are and messing with the formula unless absolutely necessary isn't really an option. Fortunately I was given a prescription for anti-nausea medication that eliminated the sour stomach symptoms so I could eat. Without the Promethazine anti-nausea meds I probably couldn't have completed treatment.

- A side note about Promethazine, it's an antihistamine, a class of drugs that tend to cause drowsiness. Because of my drug sensitivity I only took one of the take-one-or-two-every-six-hour option stated on the label. I downed it with dinner at five p.m., and was in bed within about forty-five minutes and slept for thirteen hours straight. I am not kidding about my sensitivity to drugs. I ended up taking one quarter of a pill with each meal and that was sufficient to get me through treatment. But even that small a dosage still made me drowsy. I took lots of naps. My digestion is better now but I still have to be careful not to tax my liver by eating too late in the day or eating heavy food. I love ice cream but my liver does not.

For those with challenged digestion you may want to consider some of the following information/tips:

- Dairy products except for yogurt and similar cultured milk products are a lot of work for the body to break down, especially cheese. Try to cut down on your dairy product intake as much as possible. Feta is a good alternative to regular cow's milk cheese. String cheese and mozzarella with their low fat content are easier to digest as well.

- Oil, likewise, is a heavy food. A couple of healthy oils are olive oil and flax seed oil. They are best if not heated; use them in salad with lemon juice or even on bread instead of butter. Coconut oil is another healthy alternative and can be used cold or heated for cooking. Try to avoid fried foods, especially deep frying. French fries are not a liver friendly food. I eat them about once a year and call it good.

- You can cook meat of any kind on a bed of onions without oil, or bake it in the oven.

- Ginger is very good for aiding digestion. I used fresh grated ginger and added it to tea, salad, soup, or just about anything you can imagine. If you're not used to fresh ginger start with small amounts, it can be strong for some folks. Trader Joe's ginger chews made by Ginger People were a life saver during treatment when I wanted something sweet but didn't have much of an appetite. They're a bit hot but very satisfying and good for you.

- I have to put a plug in for one of my favorite healthy habits here, fresh vegetable juice. Tons of nutrition with hardly any digestion, what a treat for your liver. You'll need to invest in a juicer (go online and do a little research) which you can get for about $75 to $100. Don't get a really cheap one because they are usually not very durable. Juicers fall into the category of things that people buy and then don't use much, like exercise equipment, so getting a used one can be a good way to save money and try it out. Juicing is a bit of work, but well worth the effort, and once you make it a habit it's a breeze. When you first start making your own juice go slow and work on your combinations carefully so you get used to the taste and don't make a big glass of something you don't like. Straight carrot or carrot and apple juice is a good way to start. A word of caution, if you include beets in your juice mix it can make it look like you have a bloody stool the next day. I just couldn't leave you to that possible freak-out without a heads up.

- My daily juice blend: The base is carrots and an apple or two. From there you can add other things; I usually throw in about an inch long piece of ginger (that's a lot by the way) along with about a quarter to half of a beet (depending on size) and two or three stalks of celery. Go online or get a book on juicing for more info. I also add a scoop of my favorite green drink powder to really kick it into gear. Drink it within about five minutes because fresh juice will oxidize quickly and lose its nutrition. Carrot juice from the store, even a health food store isn't a good substitute because it's been pasteurized. It will taste good, but most if not all of the nutrition will be lost from the pasteurizing process. But it is a good way to at least see what fresh carrot juice tastes like if you've never had it, it's very sweet. After my first taste of carrot juice I was hooked.

- You can cut down on a lot of work by just scrubbing the fruits and veggies with a brush and water to clean them. Don't peel because you will lose a lot of vitamins and nutrients if you do. Don't core apples the juicer will sort out seeds.

- Be sure to use organic carrots and other fruits and veggies if available. Besides the obvious health benefits, they taste much better. It's an unfortunate fact of mass food production that tons of pesticides, herbicides, and chemical fertilizers are loading our stores with food that's hardly fit to eat and provides very little nutrition. Keep in mind that all those pesticides/herbicides and other such toxics will need to be filtered through your liver.

Special note for Incivek users in the triple-therapy program. Incivek needs to be taken with a snack or meal consisting of at least twenty grams of fat to be its most effective (and you don't want to mess around with anything that will inhibit the maximum benefit of anything in this program). It is recommended that you eat twenty to thirty minutes before taking your dose.

Courtesy of HCVadvocate.org, here is a comprehensive list of what twenty grams of fat looks like. Obviously there are a lot of foods that contain fats that are not very nutritious such as potato chips and doughnuts. That type of fat is difficult for the liver to process. Keep in mind that taste can change during treatment and sometimes when you don't feel like eating much anyway, it takes just the right food to coax your taste buds. With that in mind don't go out and buy a bunch of special "fat" food to take with your meds. Try some different foods to see what works first before heading to the warehouse discount store and buying a large industrial size container of peanut butter.

Each of the following contains approximately twenty grams of fat.

- avocado – 1 cup (about 2 medium or 3 small)
- bacon – 4 slices regular
- butter – 2 tablespoons
- cheese, hard, such as cheddar, jack, Swiss, etc. – 2 oz
- cheese, soft, such as blue, camembert, goat, etc. – 2.5-3 oz
- chocolate, dark – 2 oz
- coconut, dried – 1 cup
- cooking oil (olive and coconut are among the healthiest; canola, sunflower, soy, and safflower are other healthy oils) – 1.5 tablespoons
- cream cheese, full-fat (not low fat)– 2 oz
- croissants – 2 medium
- eggnog – 2 cups
- eggs with yolks – 4 large
- flax seed oil – 1.5 tablespoons
- hamburger patty (80% lean/20% fat) – 4 oz
- ice cream – 1.5 cups
- Italian salad dressing – 5 tablespoons
- mayonnaise – 4 tablespoons
- milk, whole – 2.5 cups
- milkshake – 12 oz
- nuts such as almonds, walnuts, pistachios – 1/3 cup
- olives – 50 medium

- omelet – 2 large eggs, 1 oz cheese, cooked in 1 teaspoon of butter
- peanut butter, almond butter, etc. – 2.5 tablespoons
- pizza – 2 slices
- roasted chicken with skin – 5-6 oz
- salmon – 6 oz
- sardines in oil – 6 oz
- sour cream – ½ cup
- Starbucks Café Mocha w/whipped cream – Any grande or venti size made with whole milk and whipped cream
- sunflower seeds – 1/3 cup
- trail mix – ½ cup
- tuna salad – 3 oz with 1 tablespoon of mayo
- yogurt, whole milk – 2.5 cups (most yogurt is low or non-fat, so check)

Irritation and anger/ emotional imbalance: This is a topic that needs to be understood and paid attention to. We all know we get cranky when we don't feel well. Our nerves are on edge and our patience is in shorter supply. Many of us, me included, are not by nature the most patient of beings to start with. Feeling crummy not only heightens that impatience but also makes us less sociable and more inclined to stew in our own funky juices, so to speak. And when the juices you are stewing in are interferon, ribavirin, and now some additional hard chargers plus maybe some other drugs thrown into the mix to spice things up it can make a pretty toxic and volatile dish. We may get tired of feeling crappy and at times it can get kind of strange to the point where we don't even feel like ourselves. Our emotions and hormones are out of whack and ladies have told me that this is a good opportunity for us guys to finally get a clue of what they experience emotionally during PMS. Hey guys, when they said things like "you just don't understand," they were not kidding.

Communication, the vital element

We need to really be in touch with how we feel and try to communicate without a lot of extra irritation. It's okay to be too tired to talk or interact, we just need to say so in a kind manner and let our loved ones know ahead of time that might happen. Ask them to try to overlook when we are somewhat irritable and not react. We don't mean to be out of sorts and it's really not personal. If ever there was a time to try to communicate without tying in a lot of extra emotion this would be it. Get used to saying "sorry, I'm crabby and out of sorts, it's just this darn treatment." If people in treatment and those supporting them can keep this in mind it will make a big difference for all concerned.

Excuse me while I bite your head off

In our stressed out society we see and hear about daily examples of emotions run amuck. It's gotten to the point where road rage and like acts of public melt downs are almost common place. But the bottom line is that it's never a pretty picture and the aftermath leaves a big mess to clean up. If "normal" folks are having a hard time keeping their emotions in check there is an even greater challenge when going through treatment. It is very important to watch out for carrying things too far and getting caught up in the energy of irritation. During treatment even the most mild mannered can react in ways that are far from their normal temperament.

I can bring to mind three times in particular during my first treatment when I was ill informed and unprepared for dealing with my emotional states that I just "went off" on people verbally. All were people who are dear to my heart, my mother, my son, and my partner. In each situation I had a valid point to express and maybe even vent a little. The problem was that after I made my point and vented a little I didn't know when to stop. I was on a roll, more venting, more emotion, and more volume. I just let my emotions run away with me and used way more energy and words than were necessary. I wasn't screaming and pulling my hair out but I was giving a much larger piece of my mind than the situations called for. It's natural to feel embarrassed afterwards if we do get a little out of whack. A heartfelt apology can work wonders and let people know that you haven't totally lost your mind.

Here are a few tips to keep in mind concerning irritation and anger, and emotional states you might encounter.

- It's always a good idea to remember that people are not driving us crazy or upsetting us on purpose. Humans just are really good at doing that without a lot of conscious thought behind it. We all do it.

- Sometimes we just have to take a really deep breath, maybe a couple, and try to calm down.

- Try to tell people how you feel without having to make them responsible or feel bad for the way you feel. Try to settle for an ounce, instead of a pound of flesh!

- Emotions can easily be influenced, sometimes in a good way but other times in not so good ways. It often has more to do with how we feel rather than what is going on. And this can be very true during treatment.

- I'm one of those people who tend to wear my heart on my sleeve. But during treatment it was so weird and strange to find myself getting teary watching a touchy-feely commercial with a baby or a child in it. I wasn't just a little warm and fuzzy; I was Aunt Edna clutching a hanky watching *Gone with the Wind*. My emotional state was so over the top at times that often I would just crack up laughing at myself.

- Which brings me to the next tip; laughter truly is the best medicine. Things get goofy and a bit bizarre at times, don't try to figure it out just have a good chuckle on yourself and keep on trucking.

- If you've given someone permission to help keep you on track keep your end of the bargain by listening without going into defense/reactive mode when they try to help you.

- If you're the support person who is giving the reminder, tread lightly and try not to rub their nose in it. This is no time to get payback for anything that happened in the past. You are being entrusted with the opportunity to be a true friend, and their behavior at times might be enough to try the patience of a saint.

- Sometimes the thing we need the most when we're not feeling well is time alone, but not too alone. We all need to feel there is someone there for us even if we need the space to be on our own.

- If you've had mental health issues in the past, be sure your doctor is aware of that, and that you both keep close tabs on your mental/emotional state during treatment and for a while afterwards.

- Everyone who gets cured should get a t-shirt inscribed "I Survived Hep C & Treatment." Everyone who was a major support person should also get a t-shirt with "I Survived Supporting Someone during Hep C Treatment!"

Mild Depression: Note the word "mild," but even so, it is not to be taken lightly.

Treatment can by its very nature incline one towards depression. When you don't feel well for an extended time it's easy to feel down and funky. Some of the tips for irritation can also apply to mild depression. Even a mild depression should be shared with your doctor to be on the safe side.

Serious Depression & Suicidal thoughts and the potential for suicide: I am not qualified to venture very far into this topic and will keep my comment short. Do not try to "tough it out." Talk to your doctor or at the very least talk to a support person immediately if you are having thoughts of suicide. As stated above regarding depression, if you have a history of suicidal thoughts or attempts, stay in close touch with your doctor and therapist concerning your condition. Consider this; if people with no history of depression sometimes need to go on anti-depression meds during treatment, it means that the treatment itself has the potential to bring that out by its very nature. It is not a failure on your part, it's the drugs. Do not forget that.

Yet another perspective on side effects

Yes, HCV treatment has quite a list of potential side effects and it can be a fairly challenging program. That's why my wish for you is that you can take in this information and with the help of your doctor and a good support system come to an informed decision about your treatment. Sure, I did the conventional two-drug treatment and considering many factors of my situation it was kind of a no-brainer to make that choice once I had all the information I needed. It worked for me and so that's my personal bias from my experience. But I didn't set out to make this a book on why you should do exactly what I did. Hopefully between this information and possibly some other avenues that you have explored because of this book, or along with it, you will have a greater degree of solid ground under your feet to take a stand for your treatment as you see fit. That's the idea after all; again, one size does not fit all. And we each need to live with our own choices.

Possession by Beelzebub!

After going through HCV treatment and being cured I'm grateful for modern science and drugs that affect cures that were not available in the past. As you consider the side effects of HCV pay close attention to the reverse phenomena of minimizing side effects when you watch prescription medication commercials on TV. It's astounding to witness the glut of prescription drugs being offered in such alarming quantities these days. After the scenes of healing bliss (usually in a beautiful outdoor setting) you hear this calm matter-of-fact voice list the potential side effects: *Sudden death, rare but possible!* Many years ago SNL aired a skit that was so well done I thought at first it was really one of those allergy med commercials that are so prevalent. But as it moved through the lengthy list of possible side effects it progressively got more and more bizarre. At the point that it went from uncontrolled flatulence to possession by Beelzebub

I was rolling on the floor. But then again "sudden death" is no laughing matter either.

SECTION 11

ENDING TREATMENT

Yes, it will end

One fine day you wake up to the realization that you have completed your treatment. It's a little hard to grasp at first. There will be no interferon injection tomorrow (interferon starts each new week) and no more ribavirin, and as the case may be, no additional triple-therapy pills to take every eight hours either. The routines that have dominated your life for the past approximately six to twelve months are just gone. Actually it's a little more than hard to grasp, it's freaking astounding! Just all done!

The day following my last ribavirin dose I awoke to a bright spring day. I threw on a pair of shorts, t-shirt, and trail shoes and took a walk on the levee overlooking the small creek and miles of farmland next to where I live. It was truly a beautiful day to be alive. I thanked God, the Universe, and all who had made this incredible, crazy, challenging, and now worthwhile experience possible. I laughed out loud and my laughter turned to tears of joy and gratitude. I walked a little ways farther and pretty much repeated the whole praise, laughter, and tears thing all over again . . . several times! It just completely blew my mind that I had actually completed this "thing" that at times seemed like a bad low budget horror movie, *The Treatment that Would Never End.*

A post treatment insight

A better understanding about my own treatment and especially the side effects became clear to me a few days after my treatment was completed and I could once again see the world with some clarity and a sense of well-being. My epiphany was the realization that the side effects were not that terrible, but that the treatment does last a long time. It feels similar to when you are run down and out of sorts with a cold, or at the onset of the flu before it gets really bad. You feel like crap for sure but it's tolerable. You may even drag yourself to work. Treatment for me was pretty much like that, with some days not so bad and some days not so good. Not god awful bad, but just seems-like-forever long, and that's what I believe made it the most challenging for me. After awhile it can wear you down. Even up to the very end of the ordeal it was hard to relate to what feeling normal was like anymore and whether I'd ever feel not crappy again. I'd never heard anyone put it that way and it just kind of set me back on my heels. For me when it was over, I saw the whole experience summed up in the word "endurance" more than anything else.

Along with endurance I toss in "faith" because that was also a big factor for me. Once I'd done my homework and talked to knowledgeable doctors I was confident going into treatment that it would be a successful. I just had to put in the time and effort to get it done. Curing HCV is like a lot of other things in life; the desired outcome is a result of our time and effort combined with a dash of faith and no small amount of grace. And of course with HCV we throw in an arsenal of industrial strength meds just to give ourselves an edge. So far I have yet to meet anyone who went through a successful HCV treatment cure and wished they hadn't done the program. I also haven't met anyone who wasn't really glad when it was over.

The bottom line

The bottom line and good news on HCV treatment is that it is a finite program and well defined unlike many other challenging diseases as was previously pointed out. As you dutifully mark off your treatment calendar that blessed day will arrive. And when it's done and a cure has been achieved, YOU ARE DONE! A great blessing that human kind has is our inability to remember physical pain. No matter how bad anything is once it's done we kind of wonder what all the fuss was about. I've been told by women that is why they are able to give birth to more than one child.

"New Normal," take two

As the days and weeks pass after the end of treatment we find that we once again have to adjust to a "new normal." HCV changes us; we don't have much choice in that, it just happens as a result of the disease and its effect on our body. We do however have a lot to say about what we do in response to those changes. We jump into a lot of uncertainty when we start treatment and the whole new normal thing. Of course adjusting to feeling better is easier than adjusting to the various side effects of treatment but it still requires shifting our perspective and that takes a certain amount of time, patience, and understanding. Another point to consider is what is normal anyway? For each of us the answer to that question will be different. In my case the closest to normal I could muster was so long ago that it wouldn't be normal for me at my present age anyway. Since I can look back and see some affects of the virus going back to my mid-twenties, normal, as pertains to my physical well-being no longer has much meaning for me. My new normal is based on my daily practice of healthy habits. I admit there are times that I'd like to have more normal digestion, but what that usually means is eating with less attention to healthy options. I can see it as a liability or a blessing, it's my choice. There's a fair chance I'll live to a ripe old age because I can't kill myself with unhealthy eating habits, a normal luxury that many have.

Heading down the road , virus free

As I finish writing this book it's been a little over two years since the end of my treatment and I'm feeling better all the time. I've taken up dancing recently and can go pretty strong for two solid hours. Not very long ago I would be lucky to make it through one slow dance. I recently joined in a three day workshop that would have been unthinkable probably even a year ago. For me that is a strong indication my energy is getting better and the old fatigue challenge is lessening its grip on my life. There are a lot of personal mile markers that show up when all of a sudden I realize I'm doing something I haven't done in years. These are new gifts in my life, just very normal day-to-day things that most people take for granted. I take very little for granted these days, I'll tell you that.

Health is a verb

Many of you reading this will not have developed cirrhosis and you may also be a bit younger. Therefore being virus free might look a little or a lot different for you. Of course how you treat your liver and the relationship you develop with it will still be very important. Being virus free is a wonderful goal and a gift that can make a huge difference in your life both short and long term. In dealing with HCV we gain a lot of knowledge not only about the disease and our liver but also about how we are responsible for a large part of our overall health. We also come to realize how our attitude plays a substantial part in our health and wellbeing. During our education and cure we have an opportunity to learn some positive new lifestyle practices. If we choose to we can put those to good use for the rest of our lives and move forward with more hope and optimism for the future. We also know that the liver is the most regenerative organ in our body and if given loving care will bounce back quite well. Simply not having the virus to contend with will take a tremendous burden off the liver and allow it to function more efficiently and to continue the healing process. We can take the information we've learned and the adjustments we've made during treatment and decide how we might continue those practices to lead a more balanced and healthy life. Now we have choices we didn't have before and possibly some additional years to enjoy them.

Time to readjust

Your body has been a battlefield in a major war against the HCV virus. Your liver and other organs have been working overtime for years in dealing with the virus. On top of that, add in the months of heavy duty treatment meds and you realize that your body has endured a tremendous challenge. So while we're taking time to celebrate and be thankful, now is not the time to forget all we learned about our liver. Keep in mind that it will take about a month for the interferon to work through your system and about two months or longer for the ribavirin to exit. There may be some side effects for a while and depending on your age and condition of your liver in general, it's going to take a few months maybe as long as six months or longer before your body is feeling tip top. It's very important at this stage to practice some patience as you readjust. The good news is that you got rid of a long standing viral infection, no small thing. Everything else will balance out in due time. Maybe not as fast as we'd like, but in due time we will see and feel the difference. Try not to fret about the healing/recovery process, it may be rather slow. Two years later I'm still working on it . . . slowly but surely. But for this old hippy getting slowly better is a whole lot better than the alternative.

Don't stop the water

You are now in detox mode. Your body no longer needs the meds that you've taken to kill the virus so it's time to get them out of your system. Continuing to drink the same amount of water as during treatment is just as important now and for some time to come. How long? Forever if you want the optimal benefits of drinking water. Seriously, I ran across a website that has nothing to do with HCV but was explaining the health benefits of drinking water and guess what the formula was for how much water to drink? You guessed it; I was totally surprised to see that it's the same as what is recommended for treatment, half your body weight in ounces. Turns out that is what our body needs anyway, it's just crucial during treatment and for at least several months after while the drugs are being flushed out.

One treatment graduate from our support group came back after a few months and told us her tale of stopping the water regime when she'd completed a successful treatment and it was just like she was back on the meds. Not a fun experience so this is definitely something to be diligent about. Sure, it takes a little effort but now it's just a matter of continuing an established momentum.

If you must backslide; do it slowly

I say this half-jokingly because I know I've already beaten the diet and lifestyle drum rather vigorously. Just keep in mind that rich foods, fried foods, foods with a lot of dairy and a diet with a lot of salt and sugar are challenging to the liver under the best of circumstances. So jumping back into that type of diet right after treatment is not going to serve you well. If you cut down or eliminated much of those types of foods during treatment you want to go slow on reintroducing them back into your diet. It bears repeating that it would be a shame to heal your liver only to turn around and harm your heart or other organs due to poor diet.

After the elation of completion wears off

One last note since we've already covered taking it slow after ending treatment. After I completed treatment I quickly realized when the first few days of walking on air wore off that I didn't feel that great. I think what was prominent for me in the first few days of ending treatment was a huge emotional relief in having finally reached the finish line. It felt like I'd held my breath for six months and now I could breathe again. I did feel better physically as soon as I stopped taking the meds but after that initial rush of relief my body let me know that as with all things in life, there is no quick fix. As we've discussed there are a lot of dimensions involved in undergoing treatment; physical, mental, emotional, and possibly even spiritual. That pretty much covers the entire range of our human experience. The effects on some or all of those components of our being may need some time to balance out. And of course each of us experiences and processes life differently.

THE JOURNEY DURING & BEYOND TREATMENT

The Zen of HCV

Once you undertake this healing journey you may find it will test your patience, your endurance, your memory, and touch many other areas of your life. For a period of time it may seem like it has taken over and that it is the only thing going on in your life. And that may very well be true. The more you are able to embrace the challenges/changes that you encounter, the more you will learn about yourself and grow in the process. I'm a great believer that whoever or whatever is in front of us is our teacher in that moment. HCV and its treatment will definitely be in front of you, in your face much of the time, and demanding your full attention. May you embrace and learn the lessons that are brought your way, especially the hard ones, the ones you don't like and that you'd rather just have go away . . . they will lead you to your greatest strength and your truest heart.

I hope some of the following may be helpful on your journey.

- Change is invigoration to some, scary as hell for others, but ultimately necessary and inevitable for all.

- Try not to get too mental about what is going on, rest in your heart and spiritual grounding as best you are able. I posted this on a corner of my monitor screen to help remind me to be mindful of not getting stuck in my head: *If you must think, be it with the heart, for the mind is a fragile thing and prone to delusion.* This helped me keep things in perspective and chuckle when things got particularly crazy. Sometimes it might be hard to feel anything but a general yuck. Embrace feeling yucky as a condition that you understand will arise, peak, and then recede. Pretty much everything travels that trajectory; things arise, peak, and pass.

- Wanting our misery (side effects, etc.) to not arise, or to peak, and to pass faster than they are, is what causes stress, annoyance and generally makes us unhappy. We don't have to pretend to love our misery but it helps to see it for what it is, stuff that comes and stuff that goes. Fighting it tends to keep it around longer than necessary.

- Our side effects, state of mind, etc., like everything in the whole wide universe, arises, peaks, and then passes. We like it best when the unpleasant stuff passes. But it still has to arise and peak first! Kind of like "no gain without pain," which definitely applies to HCV treatment.

- Everything is changing all the time. Whatever you're feeling now will be replaced by something else in awhile. Treatment pretty much forces us to live in the moment if we allow it. We might not like the moment but it is all we really have and it will change in awhile, especially if we don't dwell on it.

- Joy may not be beating down our door; we may have to go out of our way to find it.

- And once more, when it gets really crappy, just remember, *this too shall pass*, it always does.

- In the end, I'm not sure treatment was the hardest thing I've ever done in this life, but it was the longest hard thing I ever did.

- At some point we realize it's all about acceptance. Maybe we got cured like the majority; maybe we didn't like the unfortunate minority (a very short time ago it was the other way around). Maybe we feel like a hundred bucks or maybe we're waiting to see how it's all gonna settle out. Maybe this is just part of the "package" we get in this life of ours. It all has something to teach us if we allow it.

- After it's all done we may very well wonder what all the fuss was about anyway.

- When my six month viral load came back "zero virus," it was a happy day! But what about if it doesn't come back cured, or somewhere in the process treatment doesn't work? I had that happen during my first treatment, it sucked big time, I will kid you not. Evidently it had more to teach me. And most likely I wouldn't have written this book for you if it had been over then.

PUTTING THE BOW
ON THE PACKAGE

Heart to heart

I hope this information you have valiantly labored through has given you hope for your future and a bit of encouragement for moving forward with whatever treatment you choose. I've said it before and I'll say it again, conventional treatment is a tough gig for sure, but it's a doable gig. At this point the main thing I'd share is that if you haven't had all the recommended testing done to determine the current state of liver damage, you should do so without fail. Don't be afraid, but do be informed. Once you know you have HCV that's the worst of the bad news right there. Anything else you learn, even if it's not great news, will be information you can use towards taking steps to make your life better. The purpose of this book was to get you plugged into good, reliable information and to ease your mind about what you can do for yourself. My goal was to speak as one HCV sufferer to another and in that process we sometimes need to vent a bit over the frustrating difficulty of getting good information. I hope this book will be read by doctors who can hear our concerns, so I voiced those concerns, and at times frustrations on behalf of all of us. In the end, to turn things around we all need to work together and compassionately educate each other to the best of our abilities.

I've tried to be as comprehensive as possible with information you might need for your education and decision making. Just keep in mind that as you go through the steps of your own healing, they are just that, steps. You take one step at a time. Use this material for reference as you go through your process. The three-drug treatment is still fairly new; things will come up that aren't covered here as well as the other new developments now in trial stages.

Now that you have established a solid foundation of information and understanding you should be well equipped to move forward. Now you can more readily absorb new information that will benefit your journey. And most importantly when you encounter *BS* you will see it for what it is, and not be easily swayed by the uninformed or those who would rather hold on to scare stories than take responsibility for their own health. Or better yet, that you might be the voice that says, "Hold on a minute, my friend, would you like to know what the real deal is?" Because in the absence of a concerted effort by the powers that be (the little powers that be, that is), you and I, and our brothers and sisters, are the ones who are going to make a difference in the lives of other HCV sufferers. We can be the voice of reason, and support we wish we would have had when we struggled to find reliable information. May you attain the greatest degree of wellness that you are capable of and share your blessings with others. Thank you for allowing me the opportunity of sharing this information and my story.

I will leave you with this final insight; with the combination of good reliable information, the application of our best efforts, and a lot of grace, it really does all work out!

Blessings and health to all.

RESOURCES

Online Hepatitis C Advocacy Organizations

The following websites provide an incredible scope of knowledge and resources on hepatitis C. There you can find all of the latest reports regarding current treatment options as well as information on cutting edge clinical trials and the latest developments in hepatitis C treatments. You will also find helpful links about how to navigate through insurance issues and how to get assistance if you do not have insurance.

Hepatitis C Support Project/HCV Advocate
www.hcvadvocate.org

One of the country's leading sources of hepatitis C information. The organization has over fourteen years of providing up-to-date information as well as sending trained hepatitis C specialists to conduct one day intensive trainings across the country. Many of their informational materials and brochures can be accessed online as well as ordered free of charge for personal and group use. The site also carries a large data base of active support groups throughout the nation.

For information on insurance and disability benefits click on "Benefits Column."

Caring Ambassadors
http://hepcchallenge.org

Another excellent grass roots organization that supplies up-to-date information and support.

HIV and Hepatitis
http://www.hivandhepatitis.com

This informative website focuses on providing information on HIV, Hepatitis C, and Hepatitis B and the additional challenge of co-infection between HIV and hepatitis.

www.oasiscliniconline.org

O.A.S.I.S. is a nonprofit clinic based in Oakland, CA. Under the leadership of Dr. Diana Sylvestre the organization provides many excellent published materials as well as online resources.

www.drugs.com/drug_interactions.php

A useful site for anyone taking supplements along with prescription medicine to check the compatibility of their meds. Be sure when using this information to also check with your own health provider to discuss possible interactions.

www.cdc.gov

Centers for Disease Control and Prevention. The US government's leading disease information center.

RECOMMENDED READING

Healing Hepatitis C, 2009

By Christopher Kennedy Lawford and Diana Sylvestre, MD

Though there have been many advancements in treatment since this book was published in 2009 it is still a worthwhile addition to any hepatitis C library. Mr. Lawford's personal style and willingness to share his story, warts and all, was a great inspiration to me in preparation for my second attempt at treatment as well as a guiding light for my own writing endeavor. Mr. Lawford along with Dr. Sylvestre, a pioneer in hepatitis C treatment through the O.A.S.I.S. clinic that she established, cover both the medical as well as personal aspects of living with and curing hepatitis C.

The Hepatitis C Help Book, 2007

By Misha Ruth Cohen, OMD, LAc, and Robert Gish, MD, with Kalia Doner

This is an in-depth presentation on the use of current Western medicine along with traditional Chinese herbal medicine. For those looking for a more in-depth study of combining the best of Western and Eastern medicine this is a must read.

Free From Hepatitis C, December 2011

By Lucinda K. Porter, RN

Written just over a year ago with an eye to the future, Ms. Porter writes from experience as one who has not only had personal

experience with treatment but is also a leading national speaker and educator on the subject of hepatitis C.

Don't Just Do Something, Sit There

By Sylvia Boorstein

Ms. Boorstein, a seasoned meditation teacher, takes a humorous light touch in this book as well as her many other books on the subject.

Taming Your Gremlin: A Surprisingly Simple Method for Getting Out of Your Own Way

By Rick Carson

One of my all time favorite books on dealing with that crazy mind chatter that continually nags us. This book is simple, very funny, and the methods for turning off the mind switch quite effective. A good read before and during treatment.

You Are Here: Discovering the Magic of the Present Moment

By Thich Nhat Hanh

In 1967, Martin Luther King Jr. nominated this humble monk from Viet Nam for the Nobel Peace Prize. His writing is very simple, yet profound, and of great comfort during challenging times.

Mindfulness in Plain English

By Bhante Henepola Gunaratana

An in-depth guide to Insight meditation. If you are serious about establishing a meditation practice, this book, by itself or along with group or personal instruction, can be an invaluable tool.

ABOUT THE AUTHOR

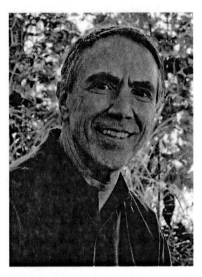

Author photo by Robert Sewell

Patrick Daniel is now free of the hepatitis C virus after a forty year journey with the illness. The same week that he completed his treatment he decided that he would write the book that he wished he would have had when he was first diagnosed. In the process he came to realize that illness, healing, writing, and reaching out to others are all part of a path and journey that is ongoing. Each step presents choices that shape our very being and spirit. And as he likes to point out, "if it was easy, it wouldn't be Earth!" With a twinkle in his eye and some hard won knowledge he offers his support wherever he can. He now divides his time between speaking and promoting HCV awareness and writing. Patrick cut his teeth on radio with a 3 hour time slot focused on HCV. He now lived outside of Sacramento, CA.

CPSIA information can be obtained at www.ICGtesting.com
Printed in the USA
LVOW11s2246140414

381730LV00011B/204/P